The Cardiovascular Disease Programme of WHO in Europe

A critical review of the
first 12 years

G. Lamm

Regional Officer for Chronic Diseases
WHO Regional Office for Europe

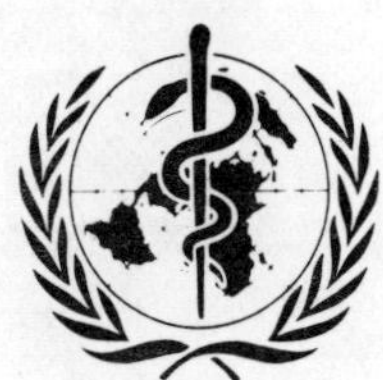

REGIONAL OFFICE FOR EUROPE
World Health Organization   Copenhagen 1981

ISBN 92 890 1151 3

PRINTED IN DENMARK

CONTENTS

1

Introduction

In 1968 the Regional Office for Europe of the World Health Organization launched a long-term programme on the study and control of cardiovascular diseases (CVD).[a] From its inception, it formed part of the worldwide CVD programme developed and coordinated since 1959 by WHO headquarters,[b] the major achievements of which have been summarized in the *WHO Chronicle (1)*.

Between 1968 and 1979, the Regional Office and WHO headquarters issued 65 reports of various working groups, two documents on consultant studies and six other major publications on various projects within the programme. Most of these summarized progress in one or another important aspect of the programme, and contained recommendations for further development. However, up to now no attempt has been made to review and analyse the European cardiovascular programme as a whole. Although years are customarily grouped in decades, a dozen years seemed an appropriate period for a summary and an assessment of the achievements and weaknesses of the programme.

The publications mentioned above contain a wealth of valuable data, accounts of methods and general guidelines. Indeed, some have become basic documents in the everyday practice of cardiology in Europe. However, the way in which they were written and presented (the Organization's "house style") sometimes made them difficult to understand, especially for readers accustomed to different kinds of medical literature. I shall therefore attempt to present here a general overview of the CVD programme as it would be written for a medical journal, limiting the use of WHO technical terms and jargon as much as possible.

This book has been written chiefly for the benefit of health professionals in fields related to cardiology (physicians, public health administrators and epidemiologists), since they are probably the people who had the greatest difficulty in comprehending the WHO reports on the programme. It is, of

---

[a] Dr Z. Pisa was at that time (1964–1973) the responsible Regional Officer; he was succeeded by the author in 1974.

[b] Dr Z. Fejfar was chief of the cardiovascular disease unit at WHO headquarters, Geneva, from 1959 to 1973.

course, very much hoped that cardiologists from all parts of Europe — many of whom assisted in the development of the programme — will also find what I have to say useful and palatable.

In a very broad and arbitrary sense, a programme in WHO consists of two major elements: (*a*) the recognition and adequate description of a problem and (*b*) the sum of actions proposed to solve it, partly or wholly. When analysing the success or failure of a programme, one might assess whether the individual actions (projects) achieved their aims, and to what extent; this may be called programme analysis, and it is relatively easy. It is much more difficult to measure the extent to which the problem itself was solved or reduced. One has to take into account not only the programme's direct, apparent effect on the problem, but also its often invisible secondary and tertiary impact — and this in the light of constant changes in socioeconomic conditions and advances in medicine. Notwithstanding these difficulties, I shall attempt to concentrate on this second kind of analysis.

2

Background

Any attempt at evaluation needs a baseline for comparison. The following is a brief review of the cardiovasular diseases situation in Europe in the 1960s, when the programme was conceived.

Clinical cardiology was thriving. The problem of rheumatic heart disease seemed to have been solved by the introduction of penicillin and the triumphs of valvular surgery. Potent new drugs had become available for the treatment of hypertension. Quickly developing new technologies providing such facilities as monitors, computers, radiography and isotopes were penetrating the cardiology departments, leading to such achievements as intensive coronary care, coronarography, bypass surgery and artificial valves, to name only a few. Apart from the appearance of these important new tools in the armoury of curative cardiology, this period was also marked by a hitherto unknown speed in disseminating new techniques. The scientific advances of the day became widespread routines in no time. Consequently, the number of cardiologists − often subspecialized in various ways − grew quickly.

Research, being inseparable from advances in clinical medicine, similarly thrived. Cardiac receptors were discovered and blocked, secrets of myocardial metabolism were uncovered, minute changes in blood-flow and their regulation were better understood, and the relation of the biophysics of the heart muscle to its function became known.

These were without doubt the golden days of cardiology, but the blaze of optimism was dimmed by the first glance at the disease statistics. Notwithstanding all the "progress" that had taken place, mortality from cardiovascular diseases − mostly coronary heart disease (CHD) − increased steadily and spread to younger age groups all over Europe. Nobody could tell whether the incidence was also rising because practically no data were available.

The menace of the CHD epidemic had already been recognized in the late 1940s in the United States. Epidemiologists were trained in cardiology and cardiologists in epidemiology; descriptive and prospective studies were launched; and differences between sexes, races, and populations were analysed. This led to the definition of a number of environmental/behavioural/biological variables suspected as being associated with the disease − the so-called risk factors. However, nowhere in Europe did advances in CVD epidemiology spread as rapidly as advances in clinical cardiology. As a discipline it was hardly recognized; those active in it could be counted on the fingers of one hand, and the idea of considering CHD as a mass phenomenon was alien to the vast majority of European cardiologists. No wonder that preventive cardiology, the direct offspring of epidemiology, slumbered undisturbed in the womb of the future. Who would dare to speak about preventing a disease the etiology of which was still unexplored? As to the modification of risk factors, that they existed at all had still not been accepted. The cardiological profession reflected, by its interest and attitudes, the picture described above. Great old men of clinical and experimental excellence "waved the flag" and shepherded the younger generation towards ever higher goals, but goals essentially very similar to their own. There were, of course, notable exceptions, but these scattered attempts to spread the new ideas of preventive cardiology were at best regarded with a quizzical academic frown.

3

The programme

A retrospective description of a programme can hardly escape endowing it with an almost perfect prospective wisdom, iron logic and unerring development. However, it must be confessed at the beginning that the CVD programme grew up organically with as many trials and errors as any living matter. The basic governing principle, however, was correct.

From the analysis of the situation it emerged clearly that if there were a role for WHO in promoting cardiology in Europe it should be towards closing the gap between the promise of clinical cardiology and the menace of increasing mortality from CVD.

The strategy of the programme was well chosen. WHO had already gained substantial recognition among cardiologists following the promotion of various research projects by the cardiovascular disease unit in Geneva. This tie with the profession was strengthened and directed slowly but deliberately towards preventive cardiology.

In the preparatory phase of the programme the lack of adequately trained personnel proved the greatest obstacle. In gradually solving this problem, the better decision was made between the alternatives. Courses and seminars were organized (or those that existed were better used) to arouse the interest of young cardiologists and give them basic training in epidemiology and preventive cardiology.

The effects of this training would have dissipated quickly had there been no "playground" provided for the newly fledged CVD epidemiologists to practise their skills. The first epidemiological surveys were begun with protocols, methods and standards (2) that had been elaborated jointly by clinicians and epidemiologists. It slowly became clear that differences in the incidence of CHD existed also in Europe, accompanied by the same risk factors as anywhere else. The first large-scale collaborative preventive trial (3) was set up. All this — and much more — happened before and during the preparations for the first long-term cardiovascular programme of the Regional Office for Europe, which was officially launched in 1968.

During the first five years of the European programme, a reasonable division of tasks was agreed on between WHO headquarters in Geneva and the Regional Office in Copenhagen, except for research which remained fully in the hands of headquarters. The worldwide problems of rheumatic heart disease, stroke and arterial hypertension were tackled from Geneva; coronary heart disease was made the main target in the European Region.

The AMI community register programme

The first major collaborative endeavour set out to elucidate two basic questions: the true impact of acute myocardial infarction (AMI) on the community, and how well existing health services match the natural history of this disease. The AMI community register programme enlisted 19 centres in Europe, one in Israel and one in Australia. Each centre represented a geographically well-defined community — a big city or an administrative part of it. Following a standard protocol, each heart attack occurring during one year in these communities was registered, and ascertained cases of AMI were followed up for one year. To answer the second question, fairly reliable data were collected about each case, concerning time of onset of symptoms, time of calling and arrival of the doctor, and time elapsed before hospitalization and beginning of coronary care. Altogether, 14 000 acute heart attacks were observed in one year (1971) in a population of 3.5 million. The attack rate varied from 7.3 per 1000 in Helsinki to 1.7 per 1000 in Sofia (Table 1). This was an important corroboration of the prevalent wide geographical differences in mortality due to coronary heart disease (Fig. 1). More shocking was the finding that despite all the advances in cardiology, which seemed likely to save many lives, the one-year mortality from AMI was still in general around 40% in the community.

The most relevant result of the study, however, was the demonstration of the discrepancy between the evolution of the attack and the availablility of medical assistance. Earlier scattered studies had demonstrated an almost 50% decrease (from 30% to 8–15%) of AMI mortality in hospital since the establishment of intensive coronary care units (CCUs). The WHO study, by covering all heart attacks, both in and out of hospital, showed that almost two thirds of the first month's mortality occurred before the patient reached hospital (Table 2). Moreover, about one third of all deaths (half of those that occurred out of hospital) happened within two hours of the first symptom. By contrast, the median time for hospitalization (i.e., the time it took half the patients to reach hospital) was 3½ hours. It thus emerged that even though coronary care units are effective, most patients in need of their life-saving interventions were dying long before they reached them. Theoretically, reducing the delay might save more lives — with the limitation, however, that a sizable proportion of deaths are sudden or occur in the first hour. Even the best services, such as that provided by mobile units, could hardly reach and assist patients in this category. A further difficulty emerged from the analysis of the details of "delay": a large part was caused by the hesitation of patients or their families to call the doctor (Fig. 2). Only 30% of patients did so within 60 minutes. Education of the public, it was thought, might help to reduce this delay, but the data failed to shown any substantial difference in such delay between first and second attacks of AMI. Little can be expected of general health education when the experience of one survived heart attack fails to change substantially the behaviour of a patient.

6

Table 1. Annual attack rate of acute myocardial infarction per 1000 population, by age and sex

	Centre	Sex	Age group (years)						Age-standardized attack rate 20–64 years[a]
			20–39	40–44	45–49	50–54	55–59	60–64	
1	Gothenburg	M	0.1	1.0	3.2	5.5	8.1	9.7	2.6
		F	0.03	0.2	0.3	0.9	2.0	3.1	0.6
2	Prague	M	0.3	1.8	3.4	7.5	11.5	12.3	3.5
		F	0.0	0.1	0.4	1.2	1.5	3.4	0.6
3	Bucharest	M	0.1	0.8	1.5	3.1	4.9	5.8	1.5
		F	0.01	0.3	0.6	0.7	1.0	2.5	0.3
4	Budapest	M	0.3	2.4	3.4	6.1	7.3	11.1	2.9
		F	0.1	0.4	0.7	1.7	1.7	4.3	0.8
6	Dublin	M	0.4	1.9	6.9	10.9	13.8	15.5	4.7
		F	0.03	0.5	1.8	2.8	3.4	5.4	1.3
7	Heidelberg	M	0.3	1.8	3.7	4.4	6.8	9.9	2.6
		F	0.02	0.1	0.3	0.4	0.7	2.3	0.4
8	Helsinki	M	0.4	4.8	9.3	14.5	21.8	26.9	7.3
		F	0.1	0.4	1.7	2.4	4.3	8.6	1.6
9	London	M	0.6	4.0	4.8	8.0	11.4	15.2	4.3
		F	0.03	1.1	1.3	1.1	3.5	5.4	1.2
10	Nijmegen	M	0.3	3.3	5.2	9.9	14.1	17.8	4.8
		F	0.1	0.5	0.4	1.3	2.4	5.7	1.0
11	Tampere	M	0.2	4.4	6.8	13.3	16.2	25.4	6.2
		F	0.0	0.0	0.7	1.9	2.6	7.1	1.1
12	Warsaw	M	0.3	2.3	3.9	5.9	8.4	10.9	3.1
		F	0.03	0.3	1.1	1.7	2.9	4.0	0.9
13	Lublin	M	0.2	2.2	3.1	5.5	7.2	9.2	2.6
		F	0.03	0.3	0.9	0.3	1.4	2.7	0.5
14	Innsbruck	M	0.2	2.0	3.7	5.6	7.3	10.2	2.8
		F	0.04	0.0	0.4	1.1	1.3	2.8	0.5
15	Kaunas	M	0.3	1.9	2.9	5.9	5.1	10.4	2.6
		F	0.0	0.2	0.3	0.8	1.2	2.4	0.4
17	Boden	M	0.2	2.6	3.3	9.0	12.7	16.0	4.1
		F	0.0	0.0	2.4	3.1	6.5	2.7	1.4
18	Sofia	M	0.2	0.8	3.2	2.3	4.2	7.0	1.7
		F	0.01	0.1	0.1	0.2	1.1	0.9	0.2
30	Perth	M	0.3	2.9	5.5	8.2	13.1	19.0	4.6
		F	0.04	0.6	1.0	2.5	4.6	6.2	1.4
31	Tel Aviv	M	0.2	2.2	4.5	6.8	8.2	19.1	3.8
		F	0.03	0.3	0.8	2.7	4.3	6.8	1.3
50	Berlin	M	0.2	1.4	3.1	3.6	9.8	8.9	2.6
		F	0.0	0.4	0.6	1.8	2.5	4.8	0.9
51	Erfurt	M	0.1	1.5	1.4	2.5	3.4	5.2	1.4
		F	0.03	0.1	0.5	0.2	1.1	0.9	0.3
52	Pasewalk	M	0.3	1.5	4.6	3.7	4.8	12.4	2.6
		F	0.0	0.0	0.0	1.1	0.7	3.8	0.5

[a] The age composition of the total population in the study areas has been used as the standard for the computation of the age-standardized rate.

8

Fig. 1. Correlation between the attack rate of AMI computed from the registers and the death rate from category 410 of the ICD (8th revision) as given in the national vital statistics: age group 55–64 years

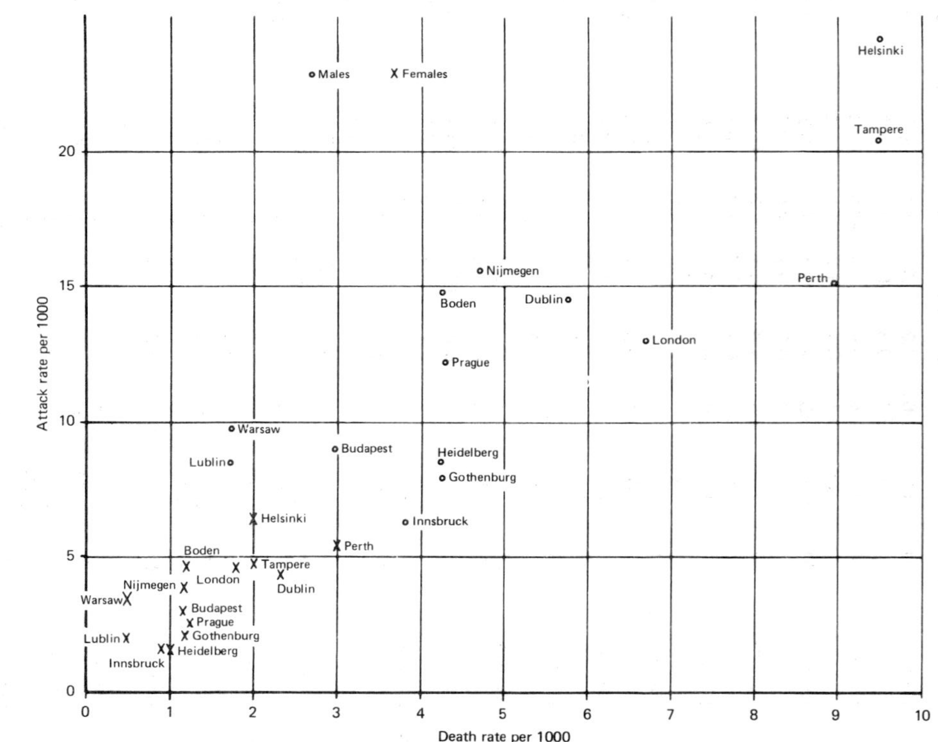

Table 2. Proportion of deaths occurring before first medical examination

Centre	Deaths within 4 weeks		Deaths within 24 hours	
	Number	Percentage occurring before first medical examination	Number	Percentage occurring before first medical examination
1	152	76	130	88
2	225	64	176	80
3	146	69	116	84
4	474	60	391	72
6	132	53	102	69
7	169	49	134	62
8	528	59	412	75
9	216	63	184	73
10	229	61	194	70
11	146	47	110	61
12	356	47	256	64
13	76	39	59	51
14	75	89	64	98
15	119	61	107	67
17	23	74	20	85
18	77	39	56	52
30	315	61	218	83
31	72	42	48	63
50	116	62	98	72
All centres	3 646	58	2 875	73

It is beyond the scope of this book to present all the results of the AMI community register study; these may be found in an earlier Regional Office publication (*4*). However, two by-products of the study merit special mention.

At the time when the medical profession refused, on ethical grounds, the idea of a randomized controlled trial for the unbiased evaluation of the merits of intensive coronary care, only about 20% of heart-attack patients were treated in a CCU. Considering that most of the registers were operating in European capitals or university towns, it may cautiously be estimated

Fig. 2. Relationship between early mortality and delays (all centres combined)

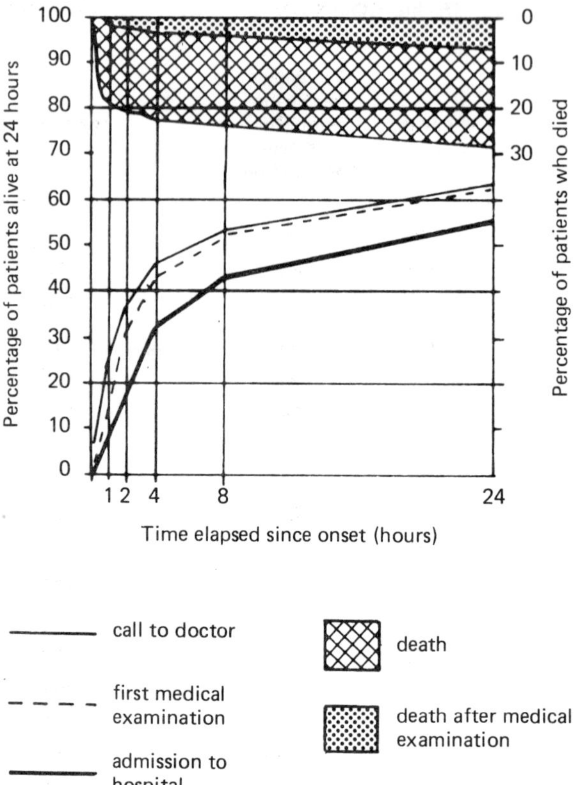

that 80–90% of the population was in fact deprived of the benefits (never properly quantified) of coronary care — although for reasons not considered to conflict with medical ethics![a]

The need for rehabilitation after AMI was also widely accepted in Europe at that time. The only question under debate was — and still is — whether it also prolonged life expectancy. However, only about one third of all registered and followed-up patients took part in a systematic rehabilitation.

These two examples show clearly that assumptions about so-called standard medical practice — based on procedures in centres of excellence — may be remote from reality.

---

[a] Even in 1975, when a number of countries were asked by the Regional Office to provide information on the number and utilization of CCUs, most of them stated that such data were not available.

When the main study ended, several centres in Europe decided to continue registration of AMI cases as a regular service. To serve this purpose, in 1974 a simplified registration system for continuous surveillance was designed (Annex 1).

It would be tempting to say that the recognition of the limitations of therapeutic intervention led directly to the focusing of attention on prevention. In fact the programme had included primary prevention of coronary heart disease much earlier.

Primary prevention of IHD using clofibrate

In 1965 an ambitious study was launched in Edinburgh to test the hypothesis that the incidence of coronary heart disease in healthy middle-aged men could be reduced by correcting their elevated serum cholesterol levels. It soon became apparent that the sample size in a single centre would be insufficient for a significant result, and WHO was asked to assist in expanding the study in Europe. On the initiative of WHO headquarters two other centres, in Budapest and Prague, joined the study. To achieve a double-blind trial (extremely difficult with dietary intervention) a lipid-lowering drug (clofibrate) was selected to achieve the immediate goal of reducing the blood cholesterol level by 15%. Fifteen thousand men were placed at random into three groups: high-cholesterol intervention, high-cholesterol placebo, and low-cholesterol placebo. The study has been described in detail (3), as well as its widely debated first results (5). It will therefore be sufficient only to highlight the main points.

In a mean treatment time of nearly six years an average cholesterol reduction of 9% was achieved, which was less than expected. Adherence to the trial was fairly good; drop-outs remained within the projected 30% throughout. The incidence of coronary heart disease ("hard-criteria" infarctions and coronary deaths) was 20% lower in the treated group than in the high-cholesterol controls. The incidence of nonfatal myocardial infarction was reduced by 25%. Both these values were significant at the 0.05 level. There was no significant difference, however, in coronary mortality between the two groups. The decrease in incidence was in full agreement with expectations based on a 9% reduction of blood cholesterol. So far, this trial could be called a success. It confirmed the hypothesis that reduction of elevated blood lipid levels, even in middled-aged men, may prevent a sizable proportion of coronary heart disease. The lack of effect on coronary deaths could be explained by the lateness of the intervention; for those with advanced disease the correction was either too small or too late, or probably both.

Unfortunately, however, the trial created more controversy than it resolved. The total number of deaths was greater in the drug-treated group than in the placebo-treated high-cholesterol control group or, after adjustment for age, the low-cholesterol controls. This excess mortality was manifested over the whole range of causes of death, thus escaping a reasonable explanation along the conventional pathways of medical logic. Owing to this alarming observation, mortality follow-up was extended well beyond the end of the trial, but even after two years of follow-up the enigma remained. Post-trial deaths showed practically the same trend as before; the difference neither disappeared

11

nor increased, no cause-specificity emerged, and no relation could be demonstrated between exposure time and mortality (6). The debate is open, with little possibility of its being resolved, over which of three tentative explanations might be correct: a "general toxic" effect of the drug, promoting death in an underlying disease; a similar vaguely defined harmful consequence of removing cholesterol from tissues; or the chance effect in the sense that, notwithstanding seemingly adequate randomization, the control group still had a fortuitously low mortality. I shall return to the problem of this trial later.

Multifactorial prevention of CHD

This monofactorial trial originated during the conception of the programme, but the European Collaborative Multifactorial Prevention Trial was a fully legitimate offspring. Initiated in 1972 in the United Kingdom and expanded to centres in Belgium, Italy, Poland and, later, Spain, this study addressed the problem of preventing coronary heart disease from a more up-to-date angle. It set out to test whether the incidence of CHD could be reduced by relatively cheap and simple methods of intervention in respect of four major risk factors: high blood pressure, smoking, high blood cholesterol levels and overweight. Instead of individuals, factories were chosen as sampling units. More than 50 similar factories were randomly assigned either to the intervention or to the control group. After initial screening, those in the top quintile of the multiple-risk score (7) were identified and exposed to intensive risk modification measures. In addition, the whole factory in the intervention group received general health education on CHD risk correction. No such attempts were made in the control factories, but mortality and morbidity were also monitored there with equal thoroughness. More than 50 000 men were finally enrolled in the trial, which lasted for six years. The United Kingdom trial has already ended, but owing to differences in times of entry to the study intervention is still going on in the other countries.

Results from the United Kingdom as regards the immediate goal, i.e. the reduction of risk factors by simple means, have already been published (8), as has interim experience from the other countries (9). These show that, with variations from country to country, multiple-risk scores were reduced by a slight to substantial degree. The final test of the success of the trial — the expected reduction in the incidence of CHD — still awaits analysis in the United Kingdom and the end of the study in the remaining countries. Until then (probably in 1982) all that can be said is that, by relatively simple means, the risk to middle-aged men can be reduced. This alone is a remarkable achievement.

Coronary care

I hinted earlier that WHO missed an opportunity to organize a proper trial for the evaluation of coronary care units (CCUs). Whether it was entirely the fault of WHO and whether it would have been possible at all at that time, remain open to speculation. However, WHO did not miss the opportunity of elaborating the basic organizational and training needs for the effective running of these CCUs in a manual (10), which has served as a guide for health departments, hospitals, cardiologists and nurses for many years. A series of working groups was convened to elucidate the special problems related to mobile coronary care units (Annex 2), to coronary care in sparsely populated areas (Annex 3), and to the inevitable problems raised by recent developments in this field (Annex 4) such as the relative merits of home care and treatment in coronary care units.

In the broader sense coronary bypass surgery belongs to the concept of coronary care, since surgical correction of the narrowed or obstructed coronary artery is care for the severely ill patient. This ingenious and often highly successful treatment spread very rapidly in the USA, the number of such operations reaching 100 000 in 1980. As in the case of other new discoveries in medicine, the need for a balanced view arose quickly — are increasing demands based on early enthusiasm and wishful thinking or on real needs? WHO attempted to resolve this problem in 1978 and a reasonable consensus was reached by setting the probable needs of bypass surgery in the neighbourhood of 400–500 per million of population — depending, of course, on the prevalence of coronary heart disease in that community (Annex 5). It should be stressed here that in most European countries even this level has not yet been reached and there is little if any evidence that Europeans are worse off because of angina pectoris than Americans.

The other problem that haunts those who advocate coronary bypass surgery is whether it prolongs life in addition to relieving symptoms. Although relief of incapacitating angina pectoris is a major achievement in itself, prolongation of life is still the ultimate value set on many medical interventions. Whether patients who have the operation live longer than those who are medically treated can be answered only by strictly controlled prospective clinical trials. With the assistance of WHO such a randomized, multicentre trial (*11*) was launched in 1973. At 12 centres in 6 countries, 768 male patients with at least 50% narrowing in two or more branches of their coronary arteries were randomly allocated to surgical and conventional medical treatment. An intermediate follow-up after two years revealed that surgical patients with three-vessel disease had significantly better survival than their medically treated colleagues (*12*). The final results are still awaited but they will probably be favourable, giving a boost to surgery in the three-vessel disease as defined. However, an early warning already seems to be warranted against claims that would extend the conclusions of this excellent study to other types of coronary patient not analysed in this trial. Furthermore, when making inferences, one has to consider the proportion of patients with three-vessel disease in the overall pool of coronary heart disease.

Rehabilitation

Developments in the rehabilitation of patients after acute myocardial infarction have been less spectacular than surgical advances but have probably had a greater effect both on patients and on the health system caring for them. In the early 1960s many experts began to challenge openly the justification for traditional treatment following AMI. Soon early mobilization became established and regular physical training was started for AMI patients, to lead them back to an active life. In close cooperation with the European Society of Cardiology, WHO fostered this new trend by providing fellowships for training in cardiac rehabilitation and later by establishing annual courses in the English, French and Russian languages.

In addition to physical exercise, new secondary preventive measures such as stopping smoking and controlling blood pressure, cholesterol levels and weight, emerged quickly. Their exact evaluation was rendered difficult by the small numbers of patients reported on in individual papers, and by a lack of diagnostic criteria and standardized procedures.

In 1970, WHO initiated a large multi-centre international study to evaluate the benefits of a comprehensive rehabilitation and secondary preventive programme following AMI, with special emphasis on discovering whether life was being prolonged by these measures (13). Twenty-three European centres and one in Israel took part in this study, for which 2700 patients were allocated randomly into intervention and conventional-care groups. Intervention focused on physical training (not necessarily supervised), cessation of smoking, control of blood pressure, dietary advice and psychosocial assistance. The intake period was rather long, the last patient being enrolled in the study in 1975. Intervention and follow-up lasted three years. The analysis focused mainly on total and cardiovascular mortality, reinfarctions, return to work and length of hospitalization. Although the study was planned as a series of national studies — owing to the wide differences between countries in attitude and socio-economic and health service systems — a centralized analysis of the major data is being attempted. Final results are expected to be available by the end of 1981. A cautious appraisal of the results at present suggests that the psychological and social benefits of this active approach are definitely not accompanied by an increase in morbidity or mortality. Some centres have shown an impressive prolongation of life in the intervention group, but this has not been confirmed in other centres. Also, up to now, institutional rehabilitation has shown no clear-cut advantage over outpatient rehabilitation.

Comprehensive control programme

At the inception of the CVD programme it was hoped that in time it would flourish into comprehensive control of CVD. This was undoubtedly very ambitious, but it was felt that the final test of each element of the programme should be its impact in reducing the incidence of the disease and alleviating the state of those still affected by it. Although the idea was there, the first step in putting it into practice was not initiated by a central decision but, as so often happens, came from the periphery. Deeply troubled by the epidemiological findings, which showed them as the world's leading community in the incidence of coronary heart disease, the people of North Karelia in Finland petitioned their government. They firmly requested concerted action to help deprive them of this unenviable world record. This happened in 1972 and marked the beginning not only of the well-known North Karelia Project (14) but also of the WHO Comprehensive Community Cardiovascular Control Programme (CCCCP) (Annex 6). This programme set out to test whether the burden of CVD in a community could be reduced by applying concomitantly, and throughout the whole community, all the established preventive and curative–rehabilitative measures for a sufficiently long time. In view of the limitations of historical comparisons (i.e., the situation before and after the programme) reference communities were also selected to be followed without intervention but with the same information system. Although differences between single pairs of intervention and reference communities might turn out to be insignificant, the trend of difference in a series of such pairs might still be conclusive.

In a nutshell, intervention included primary prevention (change of eating and smoking habits, control of hypertension, reduction of excess body weight, and promotion of physical exercise), improved care of the patient by modifying the health services, and bringing modernized rehabilitation services close to the patient. All these were innovations; the revolutionary step, however, was the participation of the whole community in the programme, beyond the boundaries of the health system. Politicians, administrators and opinion-leaders cooperated in the programme side by side with official and voluntary organizations.

Contrary to earlier attempts, the goal was to change for the better the behaviour not only of so-called high-risk groups but also that of the community as a whole. This goal was set partly because it was recognized that reversal of an already established high risk might be too late or of too little consequence, and partly because the bulk of new cases occurs with only a moderate increase in a number of risk factors, simply owing to numbers (Fig. 3). It is postulated that even a moderate reduction of the mean multiple risk will result in a substantial decline in incidence.

Registers for AMI, stroke and hypertension were set up in the pilot areas to compensate for the still inadequate information on morbidity. New methods of changing mass behaviour were designed and adapted to local conditions. Attempts went beyond imparting health knowledge, and included helping people to adopt new patterns of behaviour, e.g., by changes in food supply and price policy, the provision of outdoor and sports facilities, and legislation on smoking.

More than ten countries have joined this programme in the last seven years. Owing to the immense difficulties in launching such a complex programme — the first and decisive difficulty being to secure the commitment of communities — the programme in the pilot areas is at widely different stages of development. In some the programme is still gathering baseline information and testing the feasibility of the various elements of intervention under local conditions. In others it has closely followed the example of North Karelia and is in full swing.

Exchange of information, standardization of basic procedures, and coordination of evaluation is assisted by regular meetings of the investigators, organized by WHO. It should be emphasized, however, that this is the first project in the long-term CVD programme for which practically no seed money was needed; countries are funding the programme entirely from their own resources. The detailed report of the experience of the first five years of the North Karelia project is to be published by the WHO Regional Office for Europe (*15*) , and a brief summary has already appeared in the *British medical*

Fig. 3. Population attributable risk, based on a hypothetical population of 100 000, assuming a fourfold risk variation from 0.5% to 2.0% (the numbers of expected cases are shown inside the bars)

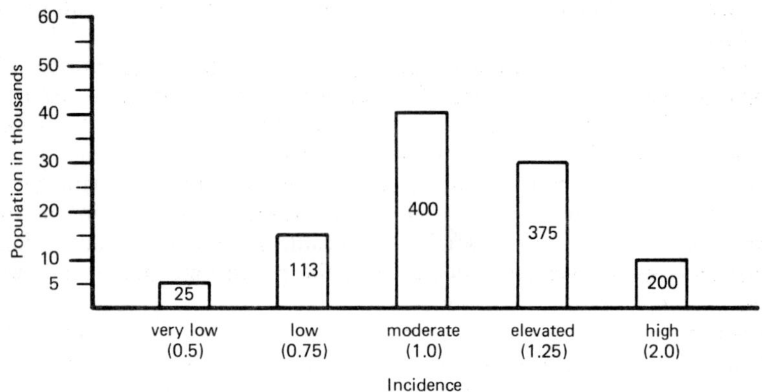

journal (*16,17*). I do not propose here to analyse the results; nevertheless, I should like to pose a personal question. Is it appropriate to evaluate, after a mere five years, a programme that set out to change lifelong habits in order to modify the outcome of a chronic disease with its origins in early childhood? A positive outcome at this stage would more befit a miracle than sound expectations.

16

4

The weaknesses of the CVD programme

It would only overburden this text to enumerate all the remaining supporting activities of the CVD programme, although their effects should not be minimized and their demands on WHO have been competing with those of the main elements described. Training, attracting experts, forging links with professional societies and national institutes, "spreading the gospel" at international conferences, etc. are examples of activities that are natural corollaries of any viable programme. Let us look instead at the weaknesses of the programme. What went wrong? What could have been done better?

It should be stressed that this section is as relevant to the assessment of the programme as the next one. It is not meant to be a witch-hunt, nor is it an exercise in masochism. I believe that we ought to publish the most conspicuous features of our internal learning process: what have we learned from our own mistakes? "Mistake" in this connotation does not necessarily mean that it *could* have been avoided under the given circumstances. It is simply to say that it *should* be avoided in the future. Others, less deeply concerned and hence possibly more objective than this writer, might add a lot to this self-criticism. Such external criticism would be most welcome.

One of the most attractive features of the long-term CVD programme was the intention to test, in a broad community, the latest achievements of cardiology while relying as much as possible on existing health services. It was hoped that positive experiences from our studies would be maintained and applied throughout the countries of the Region. Beyond this hope, however, little was done to work out a suitable timetable. The best example is the fate of the programme to establish AMI community registers. Of the 19 European registers set up, with much work and effort, 12 were not continued after the end of the official WHO programme, in 1971. We failed both in the timely planning of interesting new tasks to be performed by the registers in order to maintain local interest, and in quickly convincing central authorities of the benefits of the registers. Indeed, most of the registers that survived did so because various programmes and projects had a clear need for their data. Delay in reporting – by six years – was the main cause of the lack of enthusiastic support and expansion of the registers by central authorities. These defects in timing were aggravated by incomplete analysis of the accumulated data.

17

Many of the details of about 14 000 heart attacks were observed in a population of 3.6 million by means of the AMI register programme; 15 000 volunteers were kept under close observation (and treatment), many of them for eight years, in the Budapest–Edinburgh–Prague primary prevention trial. However, only the main results were reported descriptively rather than analytically. Analysis of the rare treasure of information available from this and other large studies is still missing. Lack of manpower and money, dwindling interest on the part of those who were engaged in the studies, and the steady accumulation of obsolescence year by year, will slowly bury these pyramids of data in the sands of oblivion. We might do well to utilize WHO research grants by inviting young scholars to analyse these centrally available data.

Reviewing the participation of countries in the programme, the list is very impressive. Most countries in Europe — and some in other regions — joined one or other activity of the programme. At the same time there were other important studies in Europe, conducted simultaneously but independently, tackling the same or closely similar problems. In most cases the reason was that some centres of excellence felt, with all justification, that they could handle the problem without associating with or relying on WHO. There is little doubt, however, that their participation would have benefited the WHO programme; in retrospect it might also have raised the value of their independent findings by providing the benefit of international comparison. For the most part, recruitment to the WHO programme took place, by necessity, through the personal contacts and acquaintances of the responsible officer in charge. While this arrangement assured that those centres that participated had the necessary skills, experience and facilities, it was far less adequate in attracting and enrolling all candidates with potential for collaboration. It might be worth while in future to adopt the system used by the National Institutes of Health in the USA whereby candidates must apply to take part in proposed research.

However, when it is borne in mind that the whole long-term CVD programme of the Regional Office was developed and managed by a single medical officer, it has to be admitted that it was a remarkable achievement. This lack of manpower was compensated for to a certain extent by the recruitment of consultants and the so-called "steering committees". The consultants assisted in the development of the various studies and trials, while the steering committees were created to guide the programme as a whole. Both mechanisms proved to be useful in assisting the regional officer to discharge the responsibilities of managing the programme. Their *ad hoc* character, i.e., one consultant for each specific task and the ever-changing composition of the steering committees, led to the lack of a stable link between the various experts and the WHO programme. We failed to set up a small body of experts having a sufficiently firm connexion with the programme and the Organization that they could contribute as much interest and creativity as the regional officer.

The direct participation of national health and research authorities was also missing. Although the programme was developed centrally, by definition, it could be executed only by devoted national experts and institutions. Their governing bodies were of course informed and gave their blessing to these activities — but in many cases no more than their blessing. Support to the national institutes concerned — in terms of both funds and broader organizational

18

assistance — came sluggishly, if at all. Often the participants in WHO studies were regarded with a certain contempt, as a foreign body among their national colleagues. In several cases the WHO emblem was much more a shield against attack than a "licence" that accorded privileges that would enhance progress. (Exceptions to this bleak picture were studies that originated in a specific country, e.g., the North Karelia project and the Edinburgh preventive trial, for which the assistance of WHO was later sought.)

All this is not to be wondered at in the absence of proper WHO mechanisms to provide transmission between national policy makers and the executors of programmes. A single-handed programme manager in Copenhagen can hardly be expected to bridge this gap everywhere.

A major achievement of the programme was the standardization of nomenclature, diagnostic criteria and methods in cardiology. When it came to specific studies, however, the standardization process exhibited many weaknesses, in spite of the abundant lip-service paid to its importance. The need for standardization was stressed, its methodology elaborated, and in certain fields facilities were even provided. The mechanism for ascertaining how far and how well these recommendations were adhered to was poorly developed. Standardization was part of the various studies and trials and not, as it should have been, a selection criterion for participating centres. Common sense and the bitter experience of the statisticians concerned with the analysis of results dictate that standardization should precede any study.

Without healthy compromises it is clearly impossible to coordinate international activities. To broaden participation or to inflate numbers, however, departures were made from the basic protocol which at the time of analysis sometimes created insoluble problems. In the study on rehabilitation and secondary prevention of AMI, for instance, individual randomization of patients was first recommended. To accommodate a few centres unable to comply, randomization of hospitals into intervention and control institutes was also accepted. Finally "randomization" of geographic areas also gained acceptance. The reader is invited to learn more about the problems thus created in the final report of the study, to be published in 1982.

The next perceived weakness is by no means characteristic only of the CVD programme, but the programme managers should have thought of it. The penetration and acceptance of WHO reports in the medical literature is very poor. Either because of the type of language in which they are written or because of the distribution system, WHO reports reach an extremely limited (and not always the best) audience. The report of the study on primary prevention of CHD by reduction of elevated cholesterol was published in the *British heart journal* and aroused worldwide interest and stimulated letters and editorials. By contrast, the similarly unique and forthright report on AMI community registers published by WHO as an independent volume in the series Public Health in Europe is seldom if ever quoted in the literature, although it reports on the largest series of AMI ever studied. The fact that nearly every published paper on AMI since 1972 (several hundred!) contains the statement "AMI was defined according to WHO criteria" — the criteria described in this very "unquoted" publication — shows that this lack of reference to WHO publications is not depreciatory or hostile; the explanation must be sought elsewhere.

Funds allocated to the programme during these twelve years show yearly contributions taking the form of a skewed Gaussian curve. Allowing for a number of external factors such as inflation, this still shows a premeditated decrease of central interest after the peak of the first few years. I feel that a curve resembling the classic haemoglobin saturation would reflect much more appropriately the funding needs of a successful programme. It is not the case that less central funding is needed when the programme is in full swing — it is simply that less is spent because no more is available. Training, quality control, consultations, exchange of personnel, and interim and final analyses are costly and by no means diminishing activities. In addition, funds granted to a programme not only have conventional purchasing power but also reflect the value and importance attached to the programme by those who have launched it. If this takes the appearance of a campaign more than that of a programme, a campaign it will be. We often call programme allotments "seed money", but any farmer knows the direct relation between the amount of seed sown and the richness of the harvest.

What has been said has more than general relevance to a long-term programme for the control of an insidiously evolving chronic disease. Length is a relative term and one may query whether even three 5-year periods may be called "long", when it comes to the control of a disease that develops over 30–40 years. Of course, there is little incentive for any one person or even an institute to engage in a difficult study, the rewards of which pour in only after four decades. There is no body other than WHO that I can think of which is better suited to engage in such studies and maintain unwavering interest and dedication for very many years, irrespective of the individuals who at one stage or another are engaged in a programme.

Last but not least comes the problem of research. The CVD programme started mainly as a series of well chosen research projects. There was never any doubt that WHO should not engage itself actively in basic research, although sometimes calls for specific basic research emanated from the Organization. Thus, the projects and studies launched in the CVD programme fell into the category of applied research, and they were called so. Few readers would disagree that the described studies of the programme were in fact research projects. (Even the most descriptive "AMI Register Study" had a null hypothesis to be refuted or confirmed, i.e., "Present care systems are well matched to the natural history of heart attacks".) With the passing of years, however, research was slowly de-emphasized in the CVD programme. Other more fashionable labels were used in the hope of attracting new mentors (and sponsors) to the programme, primarily public health administrators. The success of this change of emphasis was doubtful, and it exerted a distinctly unfavourable effect on the cardiological community. While, in the first years, many young specialists enthusiastically joined the new lines of research opened by the WHO programme, and the recognition of WHO in the professional societies grew, a new wave of alienation set in with the declared shift away from research. The rift between research in cardiology and "something" done by WHO reappeared and widened. Bear in mind that all this happened without any basic changes in the programme proper, but only as a consequence of the language used! With the decentralization of research from headquarters to the regions and the re-emerging emphasis on health research the situation is improving, but the lesson should not be forgotten — not simply for public relations reasons but for the sake of truth. New techniques in curative medicine and new hypotheses in preventive cardiology are being tested in the programme for validity and relevance. Should these two aspects not be upheld, in the light of this applied research, much misplaced work and expenditure could be saved for the health services. Confirmation, on the other hand, might not only assist health services in making better use of their limited resources, but also sometimes compel health administrations to re-evaluate health policies.

5

The achievements of the CVD programme

Some years ago when I produced a few pages along similar lines for one of our steering committees, a wise old man of international public health made the following comment: "This is all very nice. However, to convince me that these developments in cardiology are attributable, in part or *in toto,* to your activities, you should have had a control Europe — without the WHO programme!" With all the impossibility of this desideratum, the basic truth of what he said cannot be denied.

Admitting therefore from the beginning the subjectivity of this attempt, I shall still try to highlight the major steps in progress. Moreover, I shall do so without distinguishing meticulously between Regional Office and headquarters activities or even those of the European Society of Cardiology (ESC). This general approach is based on the conviction that, in as complex a problem as the overall evaluation of a large programme, it is nearly impossible to sort out cause and effect, what came first and what was secondary. Thus I leave it to the critics to challenge my statements: I generously leave it to them to produce an acceptable control Europe.

General

As a reminder let us return to the final goal of the long-term CVD programme: "To develop and test methods for the control of cardiovascular diseases in the community by relying on existing health services before their introduction for nationwide application". What was achieved in Europe in general to promote this goal?

I briefly mentioned earlier the need to train personnel for the programme, but the importance of skilled cardiologists geared to the special purposes of the programme should be emphasized again. By relying on existing training facilities, such as the courses at the London School of Hygiene and Tropical Medicine and the 10-day teaching seminars of the Council on Prevention and Epidemiology of the International Society of Cardiology (ISC), and by organizing special WHO seminars in collaboration with the Université libre de Bruxelles (1977 and 1980), several hundred young doctors underwent basic training (and had their interest aroused) in preventive cardiology. In addition, the three standard courses on statistics and epidemiology (in English, French

23

and Russian) were each injected with specific topics. Utilizing continuing studies and existing pilot areas, many individual fellowships were granted for training on the spot.

The number of people trained is a mechanical and not particularly informative indicator of effect. It is much more convincing to look through the list of people who are now engaged in promoting this new type of cardiology in Europe. More than two thirds of them took part at one time or another in these training courses. However, looking at the other side is also rewarding: about 60% of the former fellows of these courses and seminars are still engaged in activities closely related to preventive or social cardiology.

One might ask whether the consequence is direct or indirect; the fact, however, is that during the same period the number of specialized institutes and departments in Europe devoted to these problems grew substantially. Departments of cardiovascular epidemiology and prevention came into being in institutes and clinics of cardiology in, for example, the Federal Republic of Germany, Hungary, Italy, Poland, Portugal, the USSR and the United Kingdom.

The recognition and acceptance of the programme by the cardiological profession grew steadily. This rather general statement can be substantiated from four different sources. The scrutiny of the list of temporary advisers, consultants and experts associated with the programme shows a steady increase in numbers and excellence. Joint activities with the professional organizations flourished, and resulted in important publications ("How to prevent, how to rehabilitate", ISC/ESC/WHO, Vienna, 1970; "Prevention of CHD", ESC/WHO, 1978). The close tie between the Regional Office and the European Society of Cardiology was formalized in 1972; the regional officer has since been invited regularly to the meetings of its Board. Beyond this formality, at its four-yearly congresses special sessions have been reserved for reports of the WHO programme, first in Madrid in 1972 and then in Amsterdam in 1976. In 1980, in Paris, there were two such sessions. Although in Athens (1968) and in Madrid (1972) one had to look with a magnifying glass through the list of accepted papers to find a few related to the WHO programme, there was a distinct upturn in this trend in Amsterdam. In Paris, in 1980, the newly formed ESC Working Group on Epidemiology and Prevention alone presented 36 papers, and the total number of papers devoted to preventive and social cardiology amounted to over a hundred.

Recognition did not remain restricted to Europe. Although in the 1960s it seemed impossible to attain the excellence and the established standards of epidemiology and preventive cardiology of the USA, the less costly, health-service oriented approach of the programme in Europe attracted centres from other regions as well (Australia, Israel). More recently, even Canada and the USA have professed an interest in joining various parts of the programme. Another aspect that cuts through narrow regional boundaries is the use of the European experience and methods as models and incentives for the WHO worldwide CVD programme developed in Geneva, mostly for developing countries. One way to promote this is by means of the joint meetings of the principal investigators of the CCCCP programme from Europe and from the developing countries (*18*).

It was not only geographical barriers that were overcome. The character of the programme demanded an extension of reliance on expertise beyond the specialty of cardiology itself. Assistance and collaboration was sought from sociologists and behavioural scientists, through a series of working groups on health education and their direct collaboration in the pilot areas. This latter proved to be highly successful; the bulk of the achievements of the CCCCP programme can be attributed to this expertise. The attempts to prepare a fairly simple guidebook on methods of health education were much less successful. Difficulties in communication and lack of experience on both sides contributed to this meagre outcome, which hardly went beyond initiating a dialogue and establishing contacts.

It is of interest that the reverse was the case in regard to collaboration with psychologists. Joint meetings focusing on specific aspects of the programme made satisfactory progress and resulted in useful reports (*19–21*). However, great difficulties were encountered and hence relatively little progress could be made in specific programme applications, such as the elaboration of methods for psychosocial assessment, in the rehabilitation study.

The growing interest of paediatricians in problems posed in early childhood by a chronic disease of late middle age must be noted with great satisfaction. The regrettable absence of paediatric cardiologists from the spearhead of this interest can probably be explained by their preoccupation with many other acute problems.

These general — sometimes hardly perceptible — trends were reflected by more conspicuous changes. The number of countries requesting WHO advice on the establishment of new institutes or departments, or on the launching of new projects, grew steadily, and the network of WHO collaborating centres in cardiovascular diseases has grown from 6 in 1969 to 16 at the present time.

To put it briefly, the ties between WHO and the cardiology profession were strengthened, recognition grew and, a most important gain, the principles of the programme infiltrated broad sections of the health profession; this, in turn, resulted in the refertilization of the programme itself.

Specific

Epidemiology and natural history of CVD

The publication by WHO in 1968 of *Cardiovascular survey methods* (*22*) provided a firm, standard basis for conducting CVD epidemiological studies. Many such studies have been conducted since then, confirming and strengthening the evidence of large variations in the mortality and incidence of CVD — and above all coronary heart disease — in Europe. The decreasing incidence from the north-west to the south-east of Europe became well documented, although mostly from converging trends from relatively small studies rather than from several comprehensive ones with sufficiently large samples.

Differences within populations were documented, for example between different professional groups, socioeconomic classes, and religious and ethnic groups. The basic correlation between the major risk factors for coronary heart disease (age, blood pressure, cigarette smoking, cholesterol level) was corroborated. In the light of the multiple-risk theory we are now beginning to understand better the differences between the USA and Europe, and even those within Europe (e.g., France), in the changing force of individual risk factors. Clearly the population effect of cigarette smoking depends on the extent of the smoking habit in a population, and on the presence and magnitude of other risk factors (blood pressure, diet) — not to mention differences in the chemical content of tobacco.

Owing to better provision of and access to health services in Europe, the depressing picture in the USA in relation to hypertension (the halving rule along the line "existing → detected → treated → cured") did not fully apply to Europe; nevertheless, undetected and inadequately treated hypertension has been recognized as a community problem.

Wide differences in the incidence of and mortality from cerebrovascular disease were firmly established. The rates in some European countries (Bulgaria, Portugal) are almost as high as in Japan, where the toll from this disease is highest. The relation to hypertension was corroborated and some old risk factors, such as excessive consumption of salt, gained new credence in the light of recent data. The importance of transient ischaemic attacks on the brain, as precursors and indicators of stroke, was confirmed in large prospective studies (*23*).

Similarly, with regard to the natural history of the disease, the study of approximately 14 000 heart attacks in the community contributed greatly to the knowledge of limitations of existing health-service remedies.

Lastly, attention should be drawn to the emergence of new types of study. The presence and evolution of risk factors in children and adolescents are being studied with increasing frequency throughout Europe, and for preventing the development of high risk this is the most promising area in applied research in CVD.

Primary prevention

This is without doubt the most controversial issue of modern cardiology — probably even of all chronic disease specialties. There are many reasons for this, such as clinical tradition, difficulties in providing "scientific" proof, public attitudes towards health, and group and commercial interests. It seems therefore warranted to treat this subject, and WHO's contribution to its promotion, in more detail.

The story of rheumatic heart disease and especially acute rheumatic fever, though often forgotten, is in principle a good example for preventability. Except in some countries in the Mediterranean basin, rheumatic fever has ceased to be a public health problem in the last twenty years. Trends were distinctly falling well before the penicillin era, but an additional and substantial drop occurred with the introduction of systematic penicillin prophylaxis. Unfortunately — as is so often the case — few reliable data from prospective studies are available to demonstrate beyond doubt how far new preventive measures contributed to achieving and maintaining this decline in incidence. The programme on the control of rheumatic fever, run for several years by WHO headquarters in many developing countries, is trying now, with appropriate baseline data collection and standardized intervention, to fill the gap left open by countries where this information could have been gathered much more easily (*24*).

Two important conclusions are at hand. The first is that, in the absence of proper studies and an adequate information system, a disease might be "prevented" without anyone ever knowing exactly the extent of effectiveness of a particular contribution. The second is that if there are unresolved questions about the prevention of a disease of fairly established etiology, such as β-haemolytic streptococcal infection, the problem of preventing such an insidious disease as coronary heart disease or arterial hypertension, with a still unclarified but multiple causation, is obviously much greater.

The arguments for preventing coronary heart disease and arterial hypertension come from two different but amply corroborated observations. The first is that there are wide (up to eightfold) differences in the prevalence and incidence of these diseases among various populations and their subgroups. The second is that up to 60% of these differences can be explained by variations in a number of biological and behavioural characteristics, the so-called risk factors; the higher the risk levels in a population the higher the incidence, and vice versa. Conventional medical logic governed the first attempts to apply these observations for prevention. Correcting (reducing) high risk levels should decrease incidence; this philosophy is still dominant.

The three main established risk factors for coronary heart disease — high blood pressure, high serum cholesterol levels and cigarette smoking — were each attacked in the early days of the so-called monofactorial approach. WHO was no exception in joining this trend, as exemplified by the trial on the primary prevention of ischaemic heart disease by reducing elevated blood cholesterol. The blood-pressure issue was tested by a Veterans Administration study (25), and as regards the role of cigarettes the best bulk evidence — although only observational — is the experience of British doctors (26). Of course, there were many other smaller or even large studies along the same track, but the main purpose here is to present an overview.

What emerged from these studies was, in brief, partial success. It was shown that by controlling elevated blood cholestrol levels, even by pharmacological means, one can reduce the overall incidence of coronary heart disease in middle-aged males by the expected 20%; CHD mortality was not affected, however, and total mortality was higher, for reasons as yet unexplained. Control of high and moderate hypertension substantially reduced mortality due to cerebrovascular accidents and, much less convincingly, deaths from CHD. Cigarettes were clearly implicated in CHD, as well as in lung cancer, but their specific contribution to the burden of disease is still debated. There is no doubt that these studies, and WHO's part in them, contributed largely to the credibility of prevention. After the first wave of limited enthusiasm, however, a strong counter-attack emerged from various sources. Methods do not match the criteria of strict laboratory science, results are unconvincing, and their implications are unfeasible, counterproductive, even unethical — these are the main arguments of the opponents.

Before attempting to analyse this new furore, we should take a look at the so-called second-generation trial where, instead of tackling one single risk factor in isolation, the multiple-risk control approach was adopted. Allowing for the fact that the presence and level of one, two, three or more risk factors affects the incidence of the diseases not simply in an additive but in an exponential manner, these new trials attempted to correct the main risk factors simultaneously, but still in middle-aged high-risk individuals. The large study in Gothenburg, with 30 000 subjects and 10 years of intervention, has still not finished. The WHO European Collaborative Multifactorial Preventive Trial, conducted in more than 50 factories in 5 countries, has already reported success in changing favourably the overall risk profile (*9*). Corresponding data on incidence — the "final proof" — is still awaited. Similar large studies are nearing their conclusion in the USA. One particular trial — the Oslo study — has reported (*27*) a dramatic lowering of incidence in subjects selected from the top 5% of the multiple risk distribution and "treated" nearly the same way as in clinical practice (frequent visits to the same doctor, "aggressive" treatment of risky behaviour, etc.).

Again, the fully justified criticism of the inevitable weakness of these studies is tinted by crusade-like flag-waving. It is interesting that this is directed much more against proposed changes in lifestyle, such as nutrition, smoking and physical exercise, than against prevention by some kind of drug treatment, even though the impracticability and inadvisability of drug treatment at the population level is conspicuous.

There is no doubt that the pros and cons should be weighed extremely carefully before bringing about, by normative and legislative means, changes in modern "western" lifestyle. Not only are the interests of various industries and pressure groups affected, but also sometimes national or regional policies (the EEC "butter mountain"). It is no wonder that passions run high, and in their tidal wave scientific objectivity is very often washed away.

What has been shown in the last twelve years by these and numerous other studies? First, even this *a posteriori* approach (correction of high risk to reduce incidence, instead of preventing high risk from developing) has shown varying but substantial success. Second, even with relatively simple and cheap means the possibility of reversing the menacing trends of this "modern epidemic" is at hand. Third, many people are ready to comply with recommendations to change their behaviour for better health, even when these changes are not made easier for them. This being so other reasons must be sought, beyond commercial and pressure-group interests, to explain the sluggish acceptance of these findings. (Acceptance might be better in the general population than in the health profession itself!)

From the many possibilities, I should like to pinpoint only two important "mistakes". The first was overstatement. The recognition that changing eating habits together with decreasing physical exercise contributed to the increase in coronary heart disease, and that a reversal to earlier patterns might prevent to a large extent its incidence, has led to a dangerous indictment of various foods and to almost religious taboos in nutrition. Meat, butter and other dairy products have been the primary culprits in the "you shouldn't eat that . . ., avoid that . . ." gospels. Instead of explaining to people that milk is not the same as it was fifty years ago (its fat content has risen by selective breeding), that butter and cream are not natural foodstuffs but products of human manipulation, and that meat was much leaner when people themselves ate the grain that is now fed to cattle and pigs, these items were simply labelled as dangerous. Instead of teaching people how to balance their nutrition so that it

28

resembled that of their grandparents, they were given commands — what to eat, what to avoid. All this for a delayed reward, which for the individual may not even materialize! Experience shows that people are prepared to act for the sake of community health — but they have to be told to do so, openly.

The second "mistake" was overzealousness. Physically active people are, in general, healthier and this seemed to apply even to coronary heart disease. Increasing sedentariness is one of the characteristics of modern life, so let us start to run or jog (because other more entertaining and social sports facilities are lacking), especially those at high risk: late-middle-aged obese males. Although the sight of thousands of young people taking regular physical exercise in the big European cities is heartening, the increasing number of serious accidents among newly enthusiastic runners in their fifties gives ample fuel to the opponents of prevention. Similarly, the recognition that a low polyunsaturated/saturated fat ratio in the diet contributes to CHD has led to recommendations to raise this ratio, implying a polyunsaturated fatty acid consumption well above the level of the low-incidence Mediterranean countries.

After this rather lengthy description of the battlefield, are we closer to victory than we were 12 years ago?

With all their weaknesses and still unreported results, the above-mentioned studies have clearly promoted the concept of prevention. The cautious but unwavering statements in a series of WHO documents and reports (28,29) have given guidance on this controversial issue. In consequence, an increasing number of respectable professional organizations have issued statements in favour of prevention, among others the Royal College of Physicians of London, the British Cardiac Society, the Cardiology Society of the German Democratic Republic, and the European Society of Cardiology.

Action has even been taken by governments in several European countries — and not only in the form of anti-smoking legislation. Norway has laid down guidelines for new policies in nutrition for better health, which *inter alia* propose remedies for the overconsumption of calories and fats, with a compensating increase in complex carbohydrates, vegetables and fruit. Similar strong support for preventive measures has been forthcoming in Finland, the German Democratic Republic and Sweden. In the Federal Republic of Germany, a decision has been made to spend a substantial proportion of the funds allocated to research (nearly DM200 million) on problems of preventing cardiovascular diseases and cancer in the coming five years. Research in prevention is one of the main areas of coordination of the medical research council of the Council of Mutual Economic Assistance (CMEA) in the socialist countries of Europe.

For reasons mentioned earlier, even greater importance should be attached to spreading the idea of primary prevention. It has basically two new characteristics: it proposes to prevent the development of risk, instead of correcting it when it is already there, and consequently shifts the focus of interest from middle-aged high-risk people to the younger generation. The study on precursors of atherosclerosis in children conducted by WHO headquarters (Annex 7), its European ramifications, the three-centre study on possibilities of risk-factor modification in schoolchildren, and the collaborative study on the natural history of high blood pressure in children in the socialist countries are important milestones in this trend.

Summing up, we can say that the concept of promoting certain changes in health-related behaviour, which are compatible with common sense and which, according to fairly good evidence, may contribute to the decline of CHD and hypertension, is gaining acceptance. It is clear at the same time that much more research and much better information systems are needed to answer many still open questions.

Treatment and rehabilitation

"Prevention is better than cure." We have seen that the WHO programme has fully subscribed to this principle. However, no one has ever claimed the possibility of completely preventing all cardiovascular diseases. The admission that these diseases will be with us for many more centuries, if not for ever, has helped us to avoid the dangerous dichotomy between prevention and treatment.

The goals in this field have not been oriented to the promotion of new methods of treatment — this is definitely a task for basic and clinical research. The role of WHO, it was felt, should be to test the broad validity of any new treatment and to assist in disseminating knowledge of the best available therapies, not forgetting their limitations. Without reiterating the specific studies of the programme in this field, let us review how far we have succeeded in achieving these goals.

Intensive coronary care of the treatment of acute heart attacks gained quick acceptance in Europe, at least in major hospitals. Although, as shown, we failed to adhere to the logical sequence described above — first test and then disseminate — WHO guidance helped to avoid excesses. The initial zeal for overtechnicality subsided rather quickly, and the emphasis was changed to careful observation and timely intervention when the need arises. In trying to extend these coronary care units to smaller hospitals in sparsely populated areas, it turned out to be possible to achieve reasonably good results with relatively simple equipment and sensible organization of available personnel.

The demonstration of gaps between the occurrence of early deaths during heart attacks and the availability of medical aid prompted many European countries to reorganize the provisions for cardiac emergencies. Patients were encouraged to call the ambulance directly, doctors slowly abandoned going to see a heart attack patient but arranged to have them sent direct to hospital, ambulance services were reorganized, and mobile coronary care units were introduced. All this led to a substantial reduction of delay between the onset of an attack and the availability of proper treatment. Regrettably, only extrapolations can be made of the number of deaths prevented since there were no large comparative studies to assess such innovations. (One community-based study, in Budapest, demonstrated a clear reduction of early mortality, but only by historical comparison.)

Better utilization of these expensive coronary care units was achieved by reducing the time spent in them to the necessary optimum and by improvements in predictive diagnostics. As more and more experience accumulated it became apparent that many heart attacks took an uneventful course and the patients needed little medical care. This has recently led people to challenge the whole idea of intensive coronary care and even hospital treatment

30

by pointing out that most patients do well at home. This is statistically correct. Unfortunately our quick predictive diagnostic armoury has not yet developed to the stage that enables us to differentiate at the onset of the attack those who will need intensive care from those who could be treated quietly in their homes. Until it has, this claim can be substantiated on statistical and economic grounds, but it remains ethically untenable.

Although Europe is far from some leading centres in the USA (e.g., Seattle), increasing numbers of paramedical and lay people are trained in the techniques of cardiopulmonary resuscitation — another way to bridge delay until proper medical care can be begun.

Coronary care, together with the quick spread of early mobilization, has led to a substantial shortening of hospitalization for acute myocardial infarction. From what was usually 4 weeks, the period has been cut to around 2 weeks, and in some centres uncomplicated cases are sent home after 7–10 days. This, together with a 50% decrease in hospital mortality, is a remarkable achievement. Some years ago the usefulness of coronary care units was questioned on the grounds that they did not reduce overall coronary mortality. At that time, their failure to do so was clearly due partly to the lack of coverage of the whole population with coronary care unit facilities, and partly to the already mentioned mortality outside the hospital. It would be worth while to reanalyse the situation after the progress of the last five years.

Coronary bypass surgery has emerged as a major advance in the treatment of severely ill patients. The explosive growth in its use in the USA has aroused concern and led to heated debate even there. This, together with its high cost and the need for specially trained and well organized teams, has put a healthy brake on its use in Europe. Still, it was unavoidable that in certain countries the health care systems were strongly pressed to come abreast with the American level in providing this intervention, or else to bear the expense of patients being sent to the USA for their operations. Tensions rose and views clashed even in the nonmedical press.

A number of large trials have been started in the USA and, quite opportunely, also in Europe, as mentioned earlier. Most of these are concerned with whether bypass surgery prolongs life. However relevant this question is, this approach to the problem is a very narrow one. Life expectancy may remain unchanged, but the quality of life can still improve and the patient can resume normal or nearly normal daily activities. On the other hand, while prolongation of life might be proven in one subclass of CHD, as is the case in left-main disease, this cannot by implication be extended to all patients, the less so since nonsurgical treatment is also improving all the time.

There is a clear understanding that surgery, however successful, can provide a partial remedy for only a fraction of the total pool of CHD patients. Sound estimates of present and future needs have been established and are accepted in general. In this respect it should be stressed that the yearly accruing estimated need of 150 per million population will be manageable in most countries. It is only the burden of the backlog of patients in need of surgery — approximately 400 per million per year — which is inflating the number, but this is a transient demand that should disappear after a number of years. As Fig. 4 demonstrates, however, the estimated numbers of new cases per year are as yet inadequately covered in Europe and therefore the further development of bypass surgery services should be envisaged.

Fig. 4. Annual number of coronary bypass grafting (CABG) operations per million population in ten countries

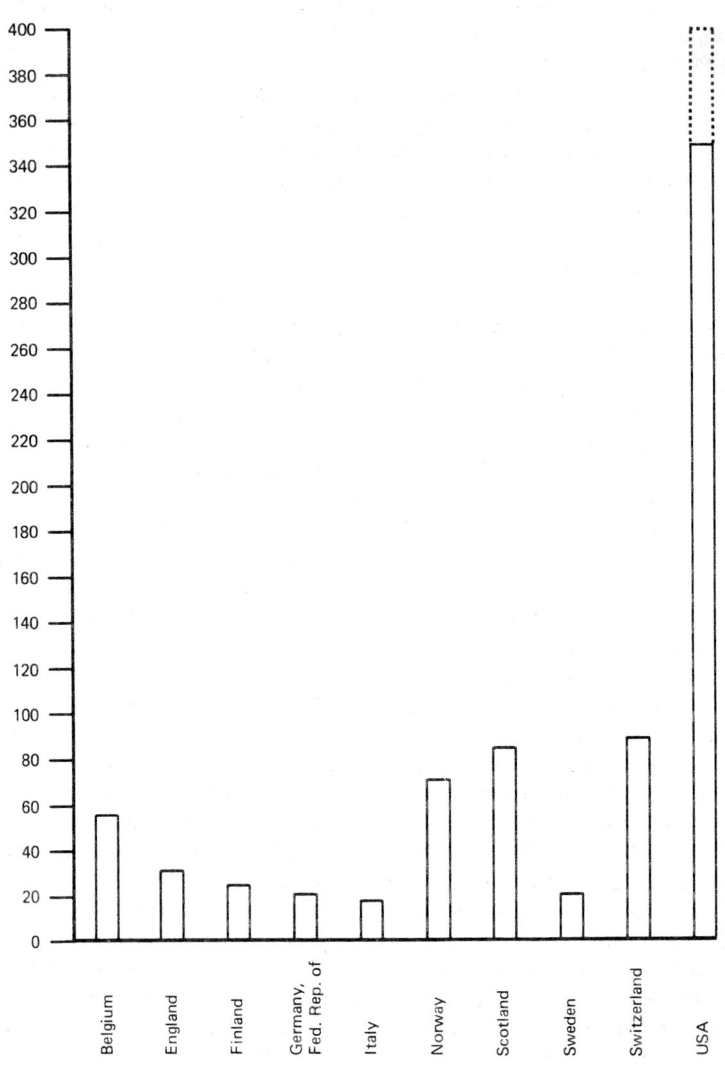

Reduction of hypertension has been the success story of pharmacology. Nevertheless, there are still in Europe many patients undetected, untreated or inadequately controlled. Although the question of defining the level of blood pressure at which treatment is more beneficial than harmful is still under study (e.g., the study on mild hypertension in the United Kingdom) the major problems in controlling clinical hypertension are mostly organizational. They involve such questions as how it should be detected and by whom, how treatment may be delivered and controlled, and how compliance may be assured. These are the well recognized problems in Europe, and this issue is discussed later in describing the WHO programme in health-care-related hypertension research.

Leaving aside many other important achievements in the treatment of CVD, for which not even an assumed influence of the WHO programme can be claimed, let us turn our attention to rehabilitation.

The progress in concept has been mentioned already. Patients after acute myocardial infarction are not regarded any longer as disabled or even handicapped victims. The large majority of them are led back to normal daily life, which includes in most cases a return to their original work. As consistent efforts and relevant studies have shown, the earlier overcautious approach to these patients did more harm than good, and it was not by any means an approach based on firm clinical or physiological foundations. Patients were "crippled" or handicapped, not because their cardiovascular system was unable to cope with the usual demands, but because they were immobilized, scared and forbidden to work (even to make love). There was not only a change in the proportion of patients making a complete recovery but also a substantial shortening of absence from work because of sickness. The period taken to return to work dropped from 6 months to 6–8 weeks in many countries, without any noticeable increase in complications or death rates. These two features are important enough in themselves, even if it cannot yet be proved that this modern approach to rehabilitation prolongs life.

Rehabilitation becomes more and more a regular part of the general treatment of the coronary patient. Institutional rehabilitation has been shown not to be a *sine qua non* of success. Indeed, the closer the links between coronary care unit and ambulatory services, the clearer it becomes that patients can be smoothly and fully rehabilitated without the inclusion of rehabilitation clinics or sanatoria. In countries where such institutions function in the conventional way, their existence can be justified by selective admission of patients, by introducing modern methods, and mainly by fitting the facilities prudently into the chain of necessary steps. Instead of providing several weeks of pleasant stay in a nice setting and contributing to the physical and psychological immobilization of the patient, they are being transformed into skilled institutions providing physical training and helping the patient to regain self-confidence and self-reliance.

Rehabilitation has been brought closer to the patient, even in rural areas, and this has shown how much the right skills with relatively little extra effort may achieve. Apart from devoted personnel — and nurses have shown themselves to be highly efficient — able to educate patients and their families and to deal with psychological and social problems as they arise, only a few well placed and well equipped outpatient clinics for the functional evaluation of heart patients are needed.

If progress continues along this line, the term "rehabilitation" could well disappear sooner or later, at least in relation to cardiology, as this activity will be incorporated in the tasks and responsibilities of normal medical practice.

6

Established knowledge and unresolved questions

Professionals and laymen alike expect firm guidance from WHO on important health problems. This expectation is warranted, as it is becoming increasingly difficult to reach a balanced view — or even to make a good decision — after being exposed to the most controversial reports and their often irreconcilable interpretations that appear in the medical literature. The normal WHO means of issuing this guidance are the expert committees, but these are convened rather infrequently. Using this opportunity, I am taking the risk of trying (*a*) to summarize for the reader what I feel are fairly well established facts that emerge from the 12-year experience of the programme, and (*b*) to make a list of still unresolved questions. This is based on interpretation of WHO reports about the programme, expert views disclosed at various meetings, and related statements of the expert committees. In spite of all this caution, however, it remains a subjective, one-man review. The same applies to the list of unresolved questions. The reader is therefore invited, if he chooses, to agree with WHO but to disagree with the author.

Are cardiovascular diseases still a major public health problem?

In 1967 CVD was the leading cause of death in Europe, accounting for roughly half of the total mortality. Half of that was due to coronary heart disease alone. The sharp decline in CVD mortality, especially that due to CHD, in the USA since 1968 triggered interest all around the world. Scrutiny of available data revealed that, except for Belgium, Finland and Norway, CHD mortality is static or continuing to rise (Table 3). This is especially evident in the younger age groups (Tables 4–6). These data are all we have and they are impressive.

It is not known, either in Europe or elsewhere, whether the decline in mortality — when it has occurred — has been due to decreased incidence, to a higher rate of cure, or to a combination of the two. Once again the lack of the right information on morbidity is evident.

Nor is there a definitive answer to the question of whether a decrease in mortality is attributable to better treatment or to progress in prevention. It is not only incidence data that are missing, but also continuous monitoring of environmental and behavioural characteristics, including the risk factors, of the population.

Table 3. Trends in coronary heart disease mortality, 1968–1977[a]

Trend	European countries	Non-European countries
Downwards	Belgium	Australia
	Finland	Canada
	Norway	Israel
		Japan
		South Africa (white population)
		United States
No change	Austria	New Zealand
	Czechoslovakia[b]	
	Germany, Federal Republic of	
	Italy	
	Netherlands	
	Switzerland	
	United Kingdom[c]	
Upwards	Bulgaria	
	Denmark	
	France	
	Hungary	
	Ireland	
	Poland	
	Romania	
	Sweden	
	Yugoslavia	

[a] From a working paper by F. Epstein for the joint Regional Office/WHO headquarters Meeting on Comprehensive Community Cardiovascular Control Programmes, Prague, 2–5 September 1980.

[b] Pending confirmation by trend analysis.

[c] Possibly a recent decline, except in Northern Ireland.

Table 4. European countries ranked in order of IHD mortality in 1975 according to category A83 of ICD-8 (deaths per 100 000; males of all ages)

Highest six[a]		Lowest six	
1.	Sweden (456)	19.	France (105)
2.	Scotland	20.	Poland
3.	Denmark	21.	Portugal
4.	England & Wales	22.	Romania
5.	Northern Ireland	23.	Yugoslavia
6.	Ireland (341)	24.	Spain (91)

[a] Finland is not among the top six countries, although it leads in the age group 35–64 years (Table 5). This is explained by the much younger age composition of the Finnish population. Note also that Sweden is at the top of the list for all ages, whereas it is not among the top six for age-specific mortality (Table 5).

Table 5. European countries ranked in order of IHD mortality in 1975 according to category A83 of ICD-8 (deaths per 100 000; males aged 35–64 years)

Ranking	Age group (years)		
	35–44	45–54	55–64
1.	Northern Ireland (81)	Finland (420)	Finland (1007)
2.	Finland	Northern Ireland	Scotland
3.	Scotland	Scotland	Northern Ireland
4.	Hungary	Ireland	Ireland
5.	Ireland	England & Wales	England & Wales
6.	England & Wales (59)	Denmark (214)	Denmark (630)

Table 6. European countries ranked in order of percentage increase in IHD mortality among males during the period 1968–1975

Ranking	Age group (years)			
	All ages	35–44	45–54	55–64
1.	Poland (65)	Poland (70)	Poland (70)	Poland (48)
2.	Germany, Fed. Rep. of	Sweden	Northern Ireland	Sweden
3.	Sweden	Hungary	Hungary	Hungary
4.	Switzerland	Denmark	Denmark	Denmark
5.	Czechoslovakia	Ireland	Ireland	Czechoslovakia
6.	Denmark (30)	Northern Ireland (11)	Czechoslovakia (25)	Ireland (6)

What is ripe for public health action and what still needs to be studied in prevention?

From the triad of preventive trials, community control programmes and increasing public interest, two general inferences can safely be made.

1. The interest of people in adopting established preventive standards in their behaviour should be aroused.

2. Changes in behaviour and lifestyle, in the direction of health promotion, should be facilitated for all those who choose to make them.

Nutrition and lifestyle

In the last 80 years technological changes in agricultural production and food processing have led not only to quantitative increases in yield but also to substantial qualitative increases in the nutritional value of foodstuffs. While few queried these changes until quantity became the main problem — as it still is in most parts of the world — the time has come to revise the health effects of those changes in affluent countries.

Calories. While it is impossible to give general optimal intake levels, it is clear that excessive intake of calories is a major problem now in most European countries. The most obvious means of control is reduction of "empty calories", i.e. refined carbohydrates and, to a certain extent, fats.

Fats. The proportion of the total calorie intake provided by fats should be kept to around 30% (in contrast to the current intake of over 40% in some countries). In particular, reduction should be aimed at saturated fats, while the contribution of polyunsaturated fats should be raised to match present levels in Mediterranean countries.

Carbohydrates. Ideally these should provide approximately 60% of caloric needs. Starchy foods are to be preferred and sugar consumption should be reduced.

Proteins. It is recommended that roughly 10% of calories come from proteins. Complete proteins, mainly from animal sources, should account for around one third of this, but more care in production, as well as pricing policies, should be devoted to keeping down the fat content of meat and milk products.

Fibre. Modern food production and "western" eating habits have reduced substantially the daily intake of fibre. Although convincing evidence for its ill effects on health is still lacking, care should be taken to stop or even to reverse this trend.

Smoking. Almost all European countries have already taken some action to curb the smoking epidemic. Its deleterious effects on health are proven, and the problem has now been moved to the field of social policy, legislation and, in some countries, agricultural–industrial readjustment.

Alcohol. Caution is warranted towards inadequately based claims that *moderate* consumption of alcohol may contribute to a lower incidence of CHD in certain populations. This claim, even if it is corroborated later, is too weak to compensate for the social, cultural, and other ill effects of alcohol consumption.

Salt. The average consumption of salt in Europe is approximately 10–15 times higher than the human physiological requirement. A sensible long-term policy should be developed to reverse this trend.

Physical activity. With rising standards of living, physical activity has decreased dramatically, although few would deny that regular, life-long exercise contributes to health in many ways. Education, city planning and promotion of socially acceptable and entertaining sports facilities for the people are sensible policies for health protection.

Blood pressure control

Better ways of identifying patients with overt hypertension should be sought, and their treatment — first hygienic, then pharmacological — should be pursued. Means of lowering the mean blood-pressure level of the whole population should be sought and tested.

There are a number of important findings on the prevention of heart diseases which merit government support for community-wide testing in pilot areas, even though their full countrywide introduction cannot be recommended as yet. These are mostly quantitative aspects of preventive principles that are already accepted qualitatively. In general, until these long-term community-wide "trials" provide further evidence of their overall benefits, it would be premature to impose the relevant behavioural changes, by legislative or other policy measures, on those who do not seek them of their own free will.

In respect of nutrition these issues include regulation of dietary cholesterol, the more exact elaboration of the optimum ratio between polyunsaturated and saturated fats, the alleged ill effects of "trans" fatty acids and overheating of polyunsaturated fatty acids, the more precise definition of quality and quantity of health-contributing fibres, and the recommendable levels of salt consumption and the Na/K ratio in food.

The levels needing treatment, the relative roles of hygienic and pharmacological intervention, and the secondary implications of life-long treatment, including side-effects of drugs, belong to the field of blood-pressure control. Basic issues such as whether to use countrywide screening for blood pressure or to adopt measures to reduce mean blood-pressure levels of populations (or their combination) can be resolved only in the light of such community-based experience.

What should be the policy towards treatment in the 1980s?

It is not possible, nor would it be reasonable to try, to cover the whole field; only the most recent developments will be dealt with.

In acute myocardial infarction the earliest contact with proper diagnostic and emergency care facilities (resuscitation, defibrillation) should be promoted. The wide availability of proper and simple assistance in the first hours after onset is to be preferred to centralized high sophistication.

Appropriate mobilization and early discharge of patients — after days, not weeks — should be pursued, followed by comprehensive rehabilitation and long-term secondary prevention integrated with primary health care. The role of special rehabilitation institutes should be defined clearly and reserved for those who gain the maximum benefit from them.

Early return to original or sheltered work should be encouraged prudently, and counterproductive social policy legislation should be reviewed in the light of new medical knowledge.

Coronary bypass surgery has proved its value for certain groups of patients suffering from medically intractable angina pectoris. According to moderate estimates, needs will show an increasing trend for a few years to come, but a reasonably manageable peak is expected in the second half of the decade. Careful decisions are constantly needed on balancing the provision of this treatment for all who really need it with the curbing of excessive demand, while bearing in mind advances in medical therapy.

Problems of hypertension treatment have already been mentioned, but it must be re-emphasized that there are still important questions about the drug treatment of so-called mild hypertension for research to clarify.

In rheumatic heart disease much can still be done to improve long-term treatment of patients with rheumatic fever (secondary prevention), especially as regards continuous monitoring of compliance and adherence to oral penicillin regimens.

The effectiveness of pacemaker treatment can be greatly raised by the use of national/regional registers and quality control systems. In calculating needs, the aging of the population and the associated spread of cardiomyopathies should not be forgotten.

What is the role of the social services in CVD control?

It seems extremely difficult to change people's behaviour, at least for health purposes. Behaviour is changing constantly under the influence of economic and political factors, and with changes in fashion. The health consequences of this changing behaviour are rarely questioned.

However, there are encouraging indications that even this difficult task may be tackled successfully. More and more, people are accepting sound advice about behavioural change *now* for future health benefits. Sometimes penetration of the population with preventive advice happens before the full backing of the health profession can be assured. (The changes in risk levels and the concomitant decline in CVD mortality in the USA may be an example.)

Much more attention should be paid to enhancing health-promoting behavioural patterns in childhood. Health education in schools should gradually be built in to various standard disciplines such as biology, environmental studies, and natural history.

Decision-makers should be in a position to initiate or promote preventive action in communities, e.g. yearly screening of blood pressure, measures that would reduce salt consumption, giving consumers the possibility of choosing "healthier" products at no more expense than other products, not only exhorting the public to avoid certain foodstuffs but seeing that alternatives are available at reasonable prices, putting hygienic considerations before commercial interests, and making roads safe for cyclists.

When communities are ready to take complex action to improve their own health, they should be encouraged and facilitated in doing so by national policy-makers.

The contribution of other disciplines such as pedagogy, psychology and sociology in health promotion should be encouraged and facilitated.

Even as regards therapy, the outcome could be greatly improved by self-reliance, improved compliance, and assistance by families, and these should be encouraged (e.g., in hypertension treatment and in rehabilitation after AMI).

The public, and the non-health social services, are not sufficiently knowledgeable about the actions they could take and the contributions they could make towards prevention. Health authorities should seek the informed contribution of agriculture and the food industry, national and local sports associations, and trade unions to the attainment of better nutrition, the promotion of physical activity, the achievement of a healthy balance between work and rest, the reduction of noise and stress, dissuasion from smoking, and other similar health-promoting actions. Voluntary organizations can do much towards assisting patients and others at risk to comply with and adhere to preventive and therapeutic regimens, and towards easing the psychosocial burden of eventual AMI-induced handicap. Patients can be guided to undertake responsibility for self-treatment — to measure their own blood pressure, for example.

7

The future

From this review of the achievements and deficiencies of the CVD programme it may be seen that CVD still is, and will remain for a long time, a major health problem. What do we intend to do about this in the coming decade?

Information

The lack of adequate information on morbidity is a common complaint in the health field, even in the computer era. It applies particularly to information on the health of populations. It is deplorable that, whenever such basic data are needed particularly urgently, a special study or project has to be undertaken to collect them.

The steady increase of coronary mortality around the world did not stimulate the establishment of adequate information systems, but its recent and hitherto unexplained decline in certain countries has provided the impetus to launch a study that will make possible the clarification of details — and, it is expected, the causes — of changes in the time trend of this disease.

Together with WHO headquarters in Geneva and the National Heart, Lung and Blood Institute at Bethesda, USA, the Regional Office has designed the draft protocol of the Monitoring System for the Incidence of CVD in the Population. The study is planned to last at least 10 years, and sets out to answer the following questions. Are changes in CVD mortality related to (*a*) improved medical care (i.e., diminishing lethality) or (*b*) decreasing incidence? If the latter, what is their relation to changes in risk factors, behaviour and socioeconomic conditions in the population?

In sufficiently large communities (of about 200 000 inhabitants), apart from the analysis of routinely available administrative data, information will be collected and validated on CVD morbidity and representative random samples will be screened repeatedly to monitor changes in risk factor levels, health-related behaviour, etc.

In addition to existing AMI registers, about 12 other centres have expressed their interest in joining this study.

One of the important concerns of the study is to attempt to stabilize the information system so that it will continue beyond the study period and

43

serve as a model for health monitoring systems in general. This implies relying as much as possible on existing structures of information and improving
their quality.

Research

The favourable consequences of decentralizing research from WHO headquarters to the Regional Offices have been mentioned briefly. One of its early
fruits is the new programme evolving in the European Regional Office on
health-care-related hypertension research.

The general role of WHO in the research field has been defined as "research coordination and promotion". Accordingly, the main purpose of the
hypertension research programme is to take stock of the national research
activities in this field, especially planned research, and to attempt to establish bilateral and multilateral collaboration among similar projects, or even
to put them under a common WHO umbrella. Thus, it differs from earlier
approaches, when WHO offered a centrally conceived programme for individual centres to join.

Medical research councils and academies from 25 European countries
participated in the first consultation on this new programme (*30*) and elaborated priority areas for joint action. Direct contacts with national research
bodies and institutions have helped to draw a fairly good picture of what is
likely to happen in the near future in Europe. It appears that, apart from
bilateral or trilateral collaboration in a number of fields, a common European programme is likely to emerge around three main problems.

1.   The natural history of high blood pressure in different populations,
environments, age groups, etc. and the role of genetic markers.

2.   Primary prevention of hypertension and its implications for health care.

3.   Treatment of the hypertensive patient (role of the general practitioner; screening or case-finding levels for, and value of, hygienic practices
and drug treatment; drug and other possible side effects of lifelong treatment; compliance, etc.).

Provision will be made for continuous updating of the information collected on research in relation to hypertension and making it available to
all potential users.

Integration

Successes and shortcomings of attempts to control single chronic diseases by
a specialized approach have led to the emergence of the idea of a more comprehensive solution. Three considerations justify this attempt.

1.   There are a number of environmental–behavioural factors which
are incriminated in the etiology of not only one chronic disease but also of

44

many others. Cigarette smoking contributes not only to CHD but also to cancer and chronic bronchitis. Nutritional factors are implicated in diabetes, cancer and gastrointestinal diseases, as well as in CVD. The list could be expanded, but the main fact is clear: there are, most probably, common risk factors for a number of chronic diseases.

2.   Single-disease-oriented programmes fail to recognize the effects of intervention on other diseases; often they repeatedly approach the same group of individuals, with only partial effects in both the collection and distribution of information (e.g., screening, health education), and the data accumulating in one specific disease programme are utilized poorly — if at all — in another chronic disease field.

3.   With health expenditure nearing its upper tolerable limits, it is becoming impossible for even the wealthiest countries to set up and operate separate specialized care services for each major chronic disease. Beyond this economic consideration it is rational to restore the unity of the patient-oriented medical approach at a higher level, rather than to continue with a single-disease-oriented approach.

The Regional Office, together with the Divison of Chronic Diseases in Geneva, is now shaping the programme, using not only the experience of the comprehensive community cardiovascular control programmes (CCCCPs) but these pilot areas themselves as starting points for a more comprehensive form of care. The first immediate goals are to establish links, cooperation and coordination among existing special chronic disease control activities in the same community, e.g., cancer and AMI registers, diabetes and CVD screening, etc. The final aim of a sensible integrated care of chronic diseases can be achieved only through an improved primary care system, where the link between various unavoidable special services is the general practitioner (*31*).

The participation of the major professional organizations has been requested. The success or failure of the programme depends mainly on the question of how far purely specialist and more general medical interests can be brought to productive harmony.

In addition, the three main areas of the CVD programme should continue, i.e., prevention, evaluation of treatment, and community control programmes. However, more national initiative, involvement, funding and even decentralized management are envisaged in these programmes. How far these expectations will be met in practice remains to be seen.

Habent sua fata libelli — and this applies to WHO programmes as well. One can only hope that as long as the problem — the burden of CVD — remains, there will always be competent and dedicated attempts to solve it in our Organization. I trust that even those who feel, after this review, that the CVD programme should have achieved much more than it has, would agree that there is still a distinct need for WHO action and leadership in respect of this disease and of a number of other chronic diseases.

REFERENCES

1. International work in cardiovascular diseases. *WHO chronicle,* **23**: 345–357, 395–404, 477–485, 524–530 (1969).
2. *Epidemiological studies on ischaemic heart disease:* reports on two Working Groups. Copenhagen, WHO Regional Office for Europe, 1969 and 1970 (documents EURO 5011(1) and EURO 5011(2)).
3. **Heady, J.A.** A cooperative trial on the primary prevention of ischaemic heart disease using clofibrate: design, methods, and progress. *Bulletin of the World Health Organization,* **48**: 243–256 (1973).
4. *Myocardial infarction community registers.* Copenhagen, WHO Regional Office for Europe, 1976 (Public Health in Europe, No. 5).
5. A co-operative trial in the primary prevention of ischaemic heart disease using clofibrate. Report from the Committee of Principal Investigators. *British heart journal,* **40**: 1069–1118 (1978).
6. W.H.O. cooperative trial on primary prevention of ischaemic heart disease using clofibrate to lower serum cholesterol: mortality follow-up. Report of the Committee of Principal Investigators. *Lancet,* **2**(8191): 379–385 (1980).
7. **World Health Organization European Collaborative Group.** An international controlled trial in the multifactorial prevention of coronary heart disease. *International journal of epidemiology,* **3**: 219–224 (1974).
8. **Rose, G. et al.** Heart disease prevention project: a randomised controlled trial in industry. *British medical journal,* No. 6216, pp. 747–751 (1980).
9. **Tunstall Pedoe, H.D.** Risk factor changes in the European multifactorial trial of prevention of CHD. *In: Proceedings of the VII ESC Congress of Cardiology, Paris, 1980.* Paris, European Society of Cardiology, 1980.
10. **Oliver, M.F. et al.** *Intensive coronary care.* Geneva, World Health Organization, 1974.
11. **Varnauskas, E. & Olsson, B.** *Progress in cardiology,* pp. 83–87 (1977).
12. **European Coronary Surgery Study Group.** Coronary-artery bypass surgery in stable angina pectoris: survival at two years. *Lancet,* **1**(8122): 889–893 (1979).
13. *Evaluation of comprehensive rehabilitative and preventive programmes for patients after acute myocardial infarction:* report on two Working Groups. Copenhagen, WHO Regional Office for Europe, 1973 (document EURO 8206(8)).
14. **Puska, P.** The North Karelia project: an attempt at community prevention of cardiovascular disease. *WHO chronicle,* **27**: 55–58 (1973).
15. **Puska, P. et al.** *The North Karelia Project: Evaluation of a comprehensive community programme for control of cardiovascular diseases in 1972–1977 in North Karelia, Finland.* Copenhagen, WHO Regional Office for Europe, 1981.
16. **Puska, P. et al.** Changes in coronary risk factors during comprehensive five-year community programme to control cardiovascular diseases (North Karelia Project). *British medical journal,* **2**: 1172–1178 (1979).

17. **Salonen, J.T. et al.** Changes in morbidity and mortality during comprehensive community programme to control cardiovascular diseases during 1972–7 in North Karelia. *British medical journal,* 2: 1178–1183 (1979).

18. *Comprehensive cardiovascular community control programme:* report of a WHO Meeting. Geneva, World Health Organization, 1979 (document CVD/79.2).

19. *Psychological aspects of the rehabilitation of cardiovascular patients:* report on a Working Group. Copenhagen, WHO Regional Office for Europe, 1970 (document EURO 5030(2)).

20. **Stocksmeier, U., ed.** *Psychological approach to the rehabilitation of coronary patients.* Berlin, Springer, 1976.

21. **Council on Rehabilitation.** *Psychological problems in cardiac rehabilitation.* Zurich, International Society of Cardiology, 1976.

22. **Rose, G.A. & Blackburn, H.** *Cardiovascular survey methods.* Geneva, World Health Organization, 1968 (Monograph Series, No. 56).

23. *Community control of stroke and hypertension:* report on a Meeting. Geneva, World Health Organization, 1974 (document CVD/74.3(II)).

24. *The community control of rheumatic fever and rheumatic heart disease:* report of a WHO Meeting. Geneva, World Health Organization, 1980 (document WHO/CVD/80.3).

25. **VA Study Group on Antihypertensive Agents.** *Journal of the American Medical Association,* **202**: 1028, 1170 (1967) and **213**: 1143 (1972); and *Circulation,* **45**: 991 (1972).

26. **Doll, R. & Hill, A.B.** Mortality in relation to smoking. *British medical journal,* **1**: 1460 (1964).

27. **Hjermann, J.** The Oslo study. *Journal of the Oslo City Hospital,* **30**: 3–17 (1980).

28. *The prevention and control of major cardiovascular diseases:* report on a Conference. Copenhagen, WHO Regional Office for Europe, 1974 (document EURO 8214).

29. **Fejfar, Z.** Prevention of cardiovascular diseases. *In: Chronic diseases.* Copenhagen, WHO Regional Office for Europe, 1973 (Public Health in Europe, No. 2), pp. 11–47.

30. *Hypertension related to health care — research priorities:* report on a WHO Consultation. Copenhagen, WHO Regional Office for Europe, 1980 (EURO Reports and Studies, No. 32).

31. *Alma-Ata 1978: Primary health care.* Geneva, World Health Organization, 1978.

A SIMPLIFIED REGISTRATION SYSTEM AND CONTINUED SURVEILLANCE OF ISCHAEMIC HEART DISEASE[a]

The Working Group on a Simplified Registration System and Continued Surveillance of Ischaemic Heart Disease, convened by the Regional Office for Europe of the World Health Organization, met in Berlin, German Democratic Republic, from 25 to 28 March 1974.

The aims of the Working Group were:

(*a*) to review and analyse the experience of those centres that had introduced simplified ischaemic heart disease registration systems;

(*b*) to discuss the future use and ways of implementing that type of service with regard to the development of community cardiovascular disease control programmes; and

(*c*) to prepare a simple model registration scheme which could be adapted to serve different local requirements.

Review of WHO ischaemic heart disease register project

In 1971 a full-scale study coordinated by WHO on registration of acute myocardial infarction in persons (both sexes) under the age of 65 years was carried out in 21 communities, of which 19 were in Europe. The preliminary results showed that it is possible to undertake a study in depth of myocardial infarction morbidity and mortality in populations of known age and sex distribution, including cases of sudden and unattended death. These studies have made it possible to compare morbidity patterns between the centres and obtain a clear picture of the natural history of acute myocardial infarction in these areas. There is, for example, a five times higher incidence of acute myocardial infarction in the Finnish and Irish centres than in Bulgaria. Furthermore, it has been found that over one third of the patients who died in the first four weeks died within the first hour of onset of symptoms and the majority of them before they had been admitted to hospital. Approximately 45% of the patients died within the first year. It is, therefore, possible to calculate that the annual incidence of heart attacks under the age of 65 years is roughly 2¼ times the annual mortality in that age group. It has also been possible to study a number of variables associated with the risk of developing ischaemic heart disease, such as weight, blood pressure and smoking habits.

---

[a] Extracted from: *A simplified registration system and continued surveillance of ischaemic heart disease:* report on a Working Group. Copenhagen, WHO Regional Office for Europe, 1974 (document EURO 8201(7)).

The registers also made it possible to study the services available for treatment and rehabilitation of patients with acute myocardial infarction. Particular note was made of the time between onset of the attack and the arrival of the doctor and of transport to hospital, of early mobilization programmes and of the cigarette smoking habits of the patient prior to the attack.

The need for continuing services and the use of a simplified scheme

Ischaemic heart disease is the most common cause of death in the European Region. In community control programmes other forms of cardiovascular disease, in particular hypertension and stroke, also have to be considered. These three disorders account for nearly half the deaths in the population of the European Region. Therefore WHO has made the control of cardiovascular diseases its major programme in its activities in Europe and has instituted similar registers to study problems of community control of stroke and hypertension.

The simplified registration scheme must be considered in conjunction with the establishment of a comprehensive cardiovascular disease community control programme, which is part of the overall programme for the control of chronic diseases.

Concept and aims of a cardiovascular disease community control programme

Favourable results from the control of rheumatic fever as a cause of acquired valvular disease, and from the surgical treatment of many congenital heart malformations in young age groups, are in striking contrast to the high incidence and prevalence of ischaemic heart disease, arterial hypertension, and cerebrovascular disease after the age of 40. At the present time there is still a lack of knowledge as far as the etiology of these three diseases is concerned. There is, on the other hand, enough evidence to show that it is possible, with proper application of scientific knowledge, to influence the disease process.

With this in mind, the WHO Regional Office for Europe has convened several working groups and meetings that have provided background information and developed methods for the implementation of cardiovascular disease control programmes on a community basis.

Cardiovascular disease control programmes are intended to reduce mortality and morbidity and help cardiovascular patients return to as normal a place as possible in the life of the community. A community in this report means a well defined, stable population.

The control of cardiovascular diseases should be achieved through comprehensive measures of intervention that have been shown to influence the natural history of the disease or are of potential use.

Intervention should be organized, and the whole cardiovascular disease community control programme should be implemented, through the existing health services in the community. In the ideal situation it could perhaps be enlarged step by step to cover a whole area or even the country.

A built-in system of evaluation is essential in any public health programme of this type. A system of registration is an operational tool to improve intervention measures and to provide information on the impact of the programme.

Present studies in simplified registration of acute myocardial infarction

A number of pilot studies on the simplified registers are at present under way. There are considerable differences between items that are collected at various centres.

In each centre the design of the register depends on the objectives for which the information is collected. The information gathered in each area depends, therefore, on the priorities in the area and they are also influenced by the resources that are available to them. The success of the registers will depend on careful planning in full cooperation with the adminstration prior to their institution.

A simplified myocardial infarction register

It was considered that the main aims of the registers were to provide:

(1) an information service for decision-makers; and

(2) an operational system for different research projects, for example:

   (*a*) prospective population studies;

   (*b*) the follow-up of acute myocardial infarction patients;

   (*c*) secondary prevention trials;

   (*d*) the endpoint for prevention trials;

   (*e*) ad hoc studies related to acute myocardial infarction.

The exact machinery to be used to collect such information will vary from country to country depending on the type of medical services and information required.

In many countries the present information systems could be used as a basis for a simplified register of heart attacks, although deficiencies do exist in such uncomplicated schemes. For instance, a number of countries undertake hospital activity analysis on a national basis, which already provides considerable information about all patients admitted to hospital. Details about those who died before admission to hospital can be obtained from the death registers, and for those who are attended by their house doctors and not admitted to hospital the social insurance schemes or national health reporting system can be utilized.

Particular attention should be given to the registration of patients below the age of 65. In the older age group there is often some doubt as to the validity of the diagnosis of acute myocardial infarction.

Review should be made six months from the onset of all registered patients, after which at least a random sample should be reviewed once a year.

An acute myocardial infarction register is an important tool for a community control programme of the disease. A comprehensive community programme may well require several registers (stroke, hypertension, etc.). For a simple ongoing register the machinery already available in the community for the collection of the required information should be used.

An acute myocardial infarction register should measure at least incidence, mortality and invalidity; in addition, it should measure certain other important indicators of the defined programme. The Group agreed on the following scheme.

Suggested items for registration in a simplified AMI register

1. *Identification of patient*
    - centre code
    - registration number or identification number
    - name and address
    - date of birth
    - sex

2. *Initial record*
    - work status prior to onset (e.g., full-time, part-time, sick leave or pension, housewife)
    - occupation group
    - criteria for diagnosis (pain, ECG, enzymes, autopsy)
    - definitive diagnosis (definite, possible, insufficient data)
    - date and time of onset
    - hospitalization (yes, no); if "yes", date and time of hospitalization
    - previous history of myocardial infarction (yes, no); if "yes", year of last episode

3. *Review record (at six months and one, two, three, four and five years)*
    - date of review
    - recovery status (normal activity, modified activity, convalescent, bedridden, dead, unknown)
    - work status (at the moment of review)
    - reinfarction since last review (yes, no)

4. *Death record (the items may be included as a part of review record)*
    - date and time of death
    - autopsy (yes, no)
    - cause of death

For the register to be a success it would appear to be necessary to have a central office and a director, who might perhaps be a cardiologist, with the final responsibility of seeing that the information is collected in the required manner. He would provide the essential link between the planners in the department of health, the register, and the doctors.

Confidentiality

WHO is aware that in some countries there is increasing concern that all personal information about an individual's health should be kept confidential; sickness registers, and especially record linkage between registers, and other information stored in data banks may provide information to administrators that the individual does not wish to be divulged. Some of this concern is spurious and is used to preserve entrenched interests, but some of it is a quite genuine fear of excessive bureaucratic control of individual freedom. In countries where such a problem is considered important by the majority, legal safeguards should be established.

Recommendations to assist in keeping the registers

1.   A training programme of personnel for information services should be organized by WHO (e.g., training courses).

2.   Definitions of terms (glossary) should be provided including specific terms used in this report, such as register, information service, etc.

3.   A further meeting would be valuable on the information services related to community control programmes using registers.

The Working Group also made the following general recommendations.

1.   Special working groups should deal with specific items, e.g., those necessary for administrators, educators and planners.

2.   Systems of data linkage should be developed.

3.   An ad hoc study on coronary care in the preclinical phase of acute myocardial infarction should be conducted.

4.   A detailed study on the medical services available to acute myocardial infarction patients should be initiated.

THE ROLE OF MOBILE CORONARY CARE UNITS[a]

The Preparatory Meeting on the Organization of Coronary Care Units, held in Copenhagen in February 1969, recommended that WHO should stimulate studies on the development of services needed to complement the work of coronary care units (CCUs) and so provide comprehensive care of acute coronary cases. While it was accepted that mobile coronary care services have saved lives, an assessment of the extent to which this has been achieved was felt necessary.

The purpose of this Working Group, therefore, was to define, on the basis of an analysis of the natural history of the heart attack, the possibilities and limitations of the mobile coronary care units (MCCUs), to review from this point of view the present experiences of MCCUs already operating in different cities in the European Region and, if found necessary, to propose a study which would help to define more precisely the contribution of the MCCUs to the care of patients with myocardial infarction (MI).

Natural history of acute myocardial infarction

The overall mortality from an acute heart attack is in the region of 40% during the first four weeks. Of all deaths during this period, at least 40% occur during the first hour, more than 50% within the first two hours, and 65% within the first twelve hours; after this time the mortality rate declines rapidly. In an as yet undetermined proportion of cases, death can be said to be instantaneous.

Because of this time distribution of deaths in myocardial infarction, a high proportion — 60% to 70% according to several studies — occur prior to hospitalization.

Mechanisms of death in acute myocardial infarction

Before the advent of coronary care units, approximately 30% of hospitalized patients died. Evidence obtained during that era suggests that one third of all deaths were due to ventricular fibrillation, approximately one third to shock, approximately one sixth to cardiac failure, and the remainder to thromboembolic events or cardiac rupture.

Ventricular fibrillation is predominantly an event of the first few hours after the onset of the symptoms. This particularly applies to "primary" ventricular

---

[a] Extracted from: *The role of mobile coronary care units:* report on a Working Group. Copenhagen, WHO Regional Office for Europe, 1970 (document EURO 5020(2)).

fibrillation (i.e., without evidence of cardiac failure or shock prior to the onset of this arrhythmia). This is relatively rare after the fourth hour following the onset of symptoms.

Ventricular fibrillation secondary to cardiac failure or shock is also commonest during the first hours but may occur at almost any time during the course of acute myocardial infarction.

Death from shock mainly occurs during the later hours of the first day and on the second and third days following acute myocardial infarction. Cardiac failure may occur at any time during the course of the attack, from the onset to two or three weeks following the first symptoms. Thromboembolic events and cardiac rupture usually occur some days after the onset but cardiac rupture is sometimes the cause of early sudden death, particularly in the elderly.

Evidence on the cause of death in the early hours of acute myocardial infarction is necessarily scanty. It seems probable, however, that most such deaths are due to ventricular fibrillation. The evidence for this is that it has been observed that most patients who die suddenly and unexpectedly in hospital do so from ventricular fibrillation. Since death from myocardial infarction outside hospital usually appears to take this sudden form, it is likely that ventricular fibrillation is the mechanism in this context also. Observations by Pantridge with the mobile coronary care unit in Belfast also suggest that ventricular fibrillation is a common cause of death in patients prior to hospital admission.

Intensive care of acute myocardial infarction

Intensive care of acute myocardial infarction is mainly directed at the prevention and treatment of arrhythmias, which cause sudden death and precipitate or aggravate cardiac failure and shock. As stated above, dangerous arrhythmias are particularly liable to develop in the first few hours after the onset of symptoms. Consequently, the sooner intensive care can be applied, the greater will be its impact.

Delay in the application of intensive care

In all communities delay exists between the onset of the disorder and the availability of the specialized staff and equipment necessary for the prevention of death, but the cause and duration of this delay differ from one community to another.

In all communities there seems to be an appreciable delay before the patient calls for medical assistance. The reasons for this include failure to recognize the significance of symptoms which may be mild, denial of symptoms, and reluctance to call for medical aid on various grounds.

In most communities, the patient calls for medical aid from a nonspecialized source. In some countries, the call goes to a general practitioner who must leave his other duties to attend to the patient. In others, the call goes to the hospital or to the general ambulance service, which sends out an ambulance staffed by a doctor and nurse, to attend to the patient. There is sometimes a delay in contacting the general practitioner or appropriate hospital department. Traffic congestion may add to the time it takes for the medical aid to reach the patient.

The attending doctor may take half an hour or more to achieve a diagnosis.

Delays during ambulance journeys occur in congested cities or when the patient has to be transported from rural areas for long distances.

Patients brought to hospital by ambulance often have to wait long periods of time whilst decisions are made about their diagnosis, management and disposal. Transport from the admission area to the CCU may also be time-consuming.

The ways in which delays may be minimized and their potential effects

There is, as yet, an undefined proportion of patients who die instantaneously or after experiencing such atypical symptoms that specialized medical aid could not be made available to them at the appropriate time. These deaths can only be prevented if the attack occurs in a place where there are persons trained in the techniques of cardiac resuscitation.

Delays in contacting medical aid could be reduced by the education of patients and potential patients. It is generally agreed that patients with known coronary artery disease should be encouraged to obtain the appropriate aid immediately they develop symptoms suggestive of myocardial infarction. Reservations are expressed about the advisability of educating the public at large in this way; it is felt that studies should be undertaken into the consequences of mass education in this subject.

The quickest method of obtaining primary medical aid appears to be by means of a centralized emergency service at which it is possible for a doctor to assess the nature of the call, and to arrange for the dispatch of the ambulance and/or the doctor nearest to the patient.

Where general practitioner services are used, availability of the general practitioner may have to be improved, or there should be alternative methods, by which he can be bypassed. It is possible in many cases for the general practitioner to make a decision with regard to admission on the telephone and thereby obviate the time taken for him to reach and assess the patient at home.

In general, delays in ambulance journeys are not great, except where there is traffic congestion or in rural areas. In remote districts, prolonged travel may be avoided by the use of aircraft or helicopters.

Delays in hospital can be diminished by improved administration in regard to admission procedures.

An important way of reducing the various types of delay is to improve, if possible, the system of communication between the various parties involved in the provision of medical care. These means of communication must be familiar to the general public.

The minimization of the delay described above, whilst enabling the more rapid admission of patients to hospital CCUs, does not bring CCU facilities to the patient at the earliest possible time – i.e., at the place of his attack. This is the purpose of the MCCU. Whilst the MCCU can ensure the most rapid application of intensive care, it can only do so if the patient's delay in seeking medical advice is also diminished or eliminated.

Mobile coronary care units

A mobile coronary care unit (MCCU) is a facility which enables personnel trained in coronary care to reach patients at the site of a heart attack (at home or elsewhere) as soon as possible, to start emergency treatment immediately, and to continue observation and treatment during transport to hospital.

Experience of MCCUs

Considerable experience of MCCUs has been obtained in Belfast, Northern Ireland and in the USSR. This has demonstrated the feasibility of operating an MCCU when it can be readily integrated with the existing system of medical organization. It has been shown that patients can be brought under intensive care much more rapidly by an MCCU than by other means and that the majority of patients can be receiving special care within two hours, and an appreciable number within one hour, of the onset of symptoms. These units have saved many lives which would have been lost from ventricular fibrillation and have been successful in preventing this and other serious arrhythmias.

Representatives from the cities in which MCCUs function have stressed the need to make general practitioners and other nonspecialized physicians aware of the importance of contacting the MCCU quickly and also of the necessity for training doctors, paramedical personnel and individuals who deal with the public in the principles of cardiac resuscitation.

Requirements that should be fulfilled before creating a mobile coronary care unit

It is agreed that mobile coronary care units are only fully effective if they are a part of an overall plan for coronary care in their area.

An MCCU must be an outgrowth of an existing and efficient hospital CCU in which the staff of the MCCU should have received training.

The way in which the MCCU actually develops must depend on the existing organization of medical services. It must supplement general practitioner services, where these exist. It is desirable that, when an MCCU is introduced into an area where no such facility has been previously known, it should be started on a pilot basis in order to test the attitude of the public and medical profession prior to full implementation.

Staffing and equipment of MCCUs

It is generally agreed that the main purpose of the MCCU is to deliver skilled medical care to the patient at the place of the attack at the earliest possible moment. It is essential for the leading member of the MCCU team to be a physician with specialized training in resuscitation, electrocardiography, anaesthetic techniques, and the diagnosis and treatment of myocardial infarction and cardiac disease in general. He should have had experience in a CCU. This doctor should be accompanied by at least one nurse who has also been trained in the techniques of coronary care. An ambulance driver is necessary, who may also help in the carrying of equipment and of the patient. Various additional personnel may be helpful.

In the cardiac ambulances in the Soviet Union, the team consists of a cardiologically-trained doctor, two paramedical workers, one of whom functions mainly as a nurse and the other who is technically trained to administer shock therapy, record ECGs, etc., and a driver. In Belfast, the team normally consists of one doctor trained in coronary care techniques, one nurse also trained in these techniques, and the driver.

It is essential that all members of the MCCU are immediately available and can be on their way to the patient within three minutes.

Unless the team can be employed in other work when they are not participating in an MCCU call, there may be under-utilization of skilled staff. In the large cities of the Soviet Union, there is usually enough work of a specialized kind to keep the cardiac teams on call employed at all times of the day and night. However, in Moscow, 9 out of 12 special cardiac teams are sometimes used for other types of emergency.

In Belfast, there is no full-time team, and the staff of the ambulance is drawn from the usual staff of the hospital. This includes members of the CCU staff and junior medical staff attached to other units who have been trained in coronary care techniques. The doctors and nurses are employed in other activities in the hospital but are able to reach the point of pick-up by the ambulance within two minutes.

Certain items of equipment are regarded as necessary for the functioning of an MCCU. These are:

- oscilloscope with ECG writer

- portable DC defibrillator

- oxygen

- apparatus for artificial ventilation, such as the Ambu apparatus (both motor-operated and hand-operated)

- laryngoscope and endotrachial tubes

- suction apparatus

- equipment for intravenous infusion and sampling

- drugs for treating pain, arrhythmias, shock and cardiac failure

Certain other equipment may be necessary in certain circumstances:

- portable battery-operated demand pacemaker with pacing electrodes

- radio telemetry, particularly when relatively inexperienced medical staff are being used, so as to permit consultation with more experienced cardiologists

- portable anaesthesia equipment when anaesthetics are used for pain relief

It should be stressed that all apparatus used under these conditions should be as compact and light as possible and that all electrical apparatus should work both from the power network and also independently (from batteries or accumulators).

MCCU facilities may be brought to the patient either in a special ambulance or in a car which is later supplemented by an ambulance suitable for transporting the patient to hospital. This ambulance must be so designed that a doctor and nurse can monitor the cardiac rhythm throughout the journey and administer treatment, including cardiac resuscitation. The ambulances in general use in some countries are suitable for this purpose; in others, a special ambulance must be obtained. One suggested way of limiting the expense of special ambulances is the use of a multipurpose ambulance. This may be appropriate for serving a multipurpose intensive care unit, but the general consensus of opinion is that, although the same vehicle may be used for a number of intensive care situations (such as cardiac arrest, respiratory failure and poisoning), the medical personnel must be specially trained for each type of emergency.

To avoid a wasteful use of ambulance drivers' time, the ambulance used for the MCCU must be based at a main ambulance depot. If this is not close to the place at which the cardiac team is located, there will be an appreciable delay whilst the team is collected. It is considered preferable, in this situation, that the team travels to the patient in a special car, followed later by an ambulance from the depot.

Inevitably, sudden deaths occur when MCCU facilities cannot be immediately available. In many cases, the affected individuals could be kept alive until the arrival of the MCCU by persons trained in first aid. It is important, therefore, that the principles and practice of cardiac resuscitation should be taught to all those likely to encounter cardiac arrest. These include, in the first place:

— doctors

— nurses

— all personnel working in hospitals

— first-aid workers

— those dealing with the public, e.g., policemen, firemen, taxi-drivers, public transport workers and those working in theatres, sports grounds, etc.

Cardiac arrest is particularly common within hospitals, often occurring outside special units or wards. It is essential that every hospital should have a mobile cardiac arrest organization with staff and equipment similar to those described for an MCCU.

Whilst it is considered desirable to interest the general public in learning about cardiac resuscitation through television and radio, it is questioned whether such media can be used effectively to teach the relevant techniques. Rather, instruction should be given to small groups so that the details of the diagnosis and management of cardiac arrest can be explained, discussed and practised. Refresher courses are needed at least annually.

Place of the mobile coronary care unit within national and regional health policy

It is recognized that the provision of MCCU facilities must take its place alongside other methods designed to promote health and provide medical care to the whole population. As discussed above, it appears that pre-hospital coronary care through MCCUs can in certain circumstances reduce mortality, but the extent of this contribution has not yet been determined for differing situations. In considering the cost-effectiveness of such units, it is important to take into account the fact that more than 30% of all deaths in middle-aged males are due to coronary disease and that more than two thirds of these deaths occur outside hospital.

It was concluded by the Preparatory Meeting on the Organization of Coronary Care Units[a] that the development of CCUs was justified in all European countries because of the high incidence in these countries of acute myocardial infarction. It was estimated that 8–10 beds would be a reasonable requirement for every 250 000 population and it was considered that the optimum size of a CCU from the operational standpoint was between 6 and 10 beds. The Working Group on MCCUs considered that where MCCU facilities were being provided, one MCCU team should be associated with one CCU for every 250 000 population. It was pointed out that, without an MCCU, uneconomic CCU facilities might develop in smaller rural hospitals; the provision of an MCCU from a larger unit might prove more economic in this situation.

It was suggested that, in addition to the system where the coronary ambulance serves a particular cardiological hospital, there might be a place for a centralized system of specialized mobile care staffed by a general city or district reserve of anti-infarct teams. It would take patients to the nearest coronary care unit where there was a free bed. This system would seem to be more effective and economic.

The experience already gained suggests that the cost is not excessive if these special ambulance and medical services can be readily integrated into the existing public health system. On the other hand, the provision of entirely separate ambulance and medical services for this purpose might well prove prohibitively expensive.

Further studies required

It is apparent that further information is needed about the human resources required to operate MCCUs, and about the impact of MCCUs on the overall mortality from acute myocardial infarction. It is considered that full data

---

[a] *The organization of coronary care units:* report on a Preparatory Meeting. Copenhagen, WHO Regional Office for Europe, 1969 (document EURO 5020).

on these questions will be available only from those centres which have registration schemes in operation prior to the introduction of MCCUs. It is therefore suggested that those centres operating registration schemes should be asked to initiate MCCU services, and to report on the results. In order to do so, information should be collected as recommended in the operating protocol for mobile coronary care units (see below).

It is also suggested that similar information should be obtained from other centres adding an MCCU to their present CCU facilities, and that the same documentation should be used in order to permit evaluation of results.

Further approaches to the problem of sudden death

As mentioned, a substantial number of sudden deaths occur under circumstances which preclude the effective application of cardiac resuscitation even when MCCUs are available. These deaths could only be prevented if they could be predicted.

It has long been recognized that patients with acute myocardial infarction, whether this presents in the classical fashion or as sudden death, have often had symptoms prior to this event. It would appear that about 50% of patients experiencing myocardial infarction or sudden death have the onset of chest pain for the first time, or exacerbation of earlier chest pains, during the days or weeks prior to the acute attack, although they do not necessarily report this to a doctor. The existence of these prodromal symptoms indicates the possible need for some intervention which might either prevent the onset of acute coronary attack or suppress its complications. Unfortunately, there are as yet no proved methods available for these purposes. Furthermore, there is no satisfactory information on how many patients develop such types of pain without proceeding to acute heart attacks, or what the median interval is between the onset of such symptoms and the acute event. Further information on this subject is essential before studies can be undertaken on the prevention and control of acute coronary attacks.

Conclusions

A mobile coronary care unit is a facility which enables personnel trained in coronary care to reach patients at the site of a heart attack (at home or elsewhere) as soon as possible, to start emergency treatment immediately, and to continue observation and treatment during transport to hospital.

Experience obtained in the USSR and in Northern Ireland has demonstrated the feasibility of operating an MCCU when this can be readily integrated with the existing system of medical organization. It has been shown that such units save lives which would otherwise have been lost, but it is still not possible to state what effects MCCUs have had, or could have, on total mortality from acute myocardial infarction in the community.

It is considered that the role of WHO in this field should be to support further studies on the human resources required to operate MCCUs and on the impact of MCCUs on the overall mortality from acute myocardial infarction.

Recommendations

1. WHO should support studies on the human resources required to operate MCCUs and on the impact of MCCUs on overall mortality from acute myocardial infarction in the centres operating registration schemes under WHO supervision.

2. When MCCUs are created, they should be organized according to the recommendations outlined on pp. 58–60. Those operating such services should be encouraged to use the documentation recommended in the operating protocol.

3. WHO should consider other approaches to solving the problem of sudden death, particularly with regard to the significance of prodromal symptoms and the management of patients with such symptoms.

Operating protocol for mobile coronary care units

The operating protocol proposed for registration areas, as included in part II of the report on the Working Group on Ischaemic Heart Disease Registers,[a] should be taken as a basis. The part dealing with the early stages of the attack should be expanded to include the following items:

Crew of ambulance:

   trained physician, nurse, medical aide

Place of onset:

   work, home, hospital

Other: place from where the call was made:

   home, public phone

Caller:

   patient, relative, witness, medical person

---

[a] *Ischaemic heart disease registers:* report on a Working Group. Copenhagen, WHO Regional Office for Europe, 1969 (document EURO 5010(2)).

Time:

    onset of symptoms[a]
    call to GP (or primary ambulance service)
    GP receives call
    GP sees the patient
    GP calls ambulance
    ambulance receives call
    ambulance starts
    arrives at place of call
    starts back
    arrives in hospital
    transfer to CCU (or medical ward)

The part dealing with the clinical condition at first medical examination should be expanded to include the following items:

    type of arrythmia, supra ventr. ES, ventr. ES, tachy, fib., lab tests, a-v block

Active management of patient:

    at home, during transport

Type of treatment:

    pacing, defibrillation, drugs — digitalis, atropine, anti-arrhythmia, blood-pressure-raising, oxygen, pain relieving, other

Cause of delay:

    administrative
    traffic congestion
    difficulty in finding the place
    difficulty in entering the house
    other

---

[a] Symptoms: chest pain, abdominal pain, fainting, breathing difficulties, palpitations, other.

CORONARY CARE OUTSIDE BIG CENTRES[a]

The Working Group on Coronary Care Outside Big Centres, convened by the Regional Office for Europe of the World Health Organization, met in Copenhagen from 4 to 6 November 1974.

This meeting was directly related to other activities of the Regional Office's long-term programme in cardiovascular diseases, particularly to the meeting held in the Regional Office in 1969 on the Organization of Coronary Care Units, and to that held in Moscow in 1970 on the Role of Mobile Coronary Care Units. The emphasis at this stage of the long-term programme is on the integration of systems of cardiovascular control into the general health services, and this is also applicable with regard to coronary care outside big centres.

Definitions

Intensive coronary care is the continuous and intensive surveillance of patients suspected of having acute myocardial infarction, in order to prevent and treat its complications, especially arrythmias. It may also include the care, under the same conditions, of other patients with acute myocardial ischaemia and of patients with serious arrhythmias not due to coronary disease.

A coronary care unit (CCU) is a self-contained unit specifically designed for intensive coronary care.

A coronary care area is an area set aside for intensive coronary care which is not self-contained but which is closely associated with an intensive care unit or medical ward.

A mobile coronary care unit (MCCU) is a facility which enables personnel trained in coronary care to reach patients at the site of a heart attack (at home or elsewhere) as soon as possible, to start emergency treatment immediately, and to continue observation and treatment during transport to hospital.

Preliminary considerations

The overall death rate in acute heart attack is in the region of 40% during the first four weeks. Of all deaths during this period, about 40% occur during the first hour, approximately 45% within the first two hours, and about 65% within the first 24 hours, but thereafter the mortality declines rapidly (Table 1). Hence, death from myocardial infarction frequently takes place

---

[a] Extracted from: *Coronary care outside big centres:* report on a Working Group. Copenhagen, WHO Regional Office for Europe, 1975 (document EURO 8204(6)).

Table 1. Mortality from acute myocardial infarction according to time elapsed between onset and death (both sexes: cases of AMI "none" excluded)

Time elapsed	Code number of centre																			All centres (average)
	01	02	03	04	06	07	08	09	10	11	12	13	14	15	17	18	30	31	50	
	%	%	%	%	%	%	%	%	%	%	%	%	%	%	%	%	%	%	%	%
Under 30 minutes	23	43	24	48	19	39	37	42	47	34	20	16	10	38	41	3	24	32	19	33
30–59 minutes	1	6	12	7	7	6	4	4	6	7	9	12	0	13	7	1	6	8	0	6
60–119 minutes	1	4	4	5	7	5	4	5	4	7	6	13	3	10	0	6	5	5	4	5
2–3 hours	4	3	4	6	3	4	4	7	6	4	5	4	6	8	0	4	3	6	6	5
4–23 hours	29	9	13	9	20	11	12	14	12	13	18	19	35	14	14	36	12	8	34	14
≥1 day	43	36	43	26	44	34	39	29	25	35	43	35	45	18	38	49	50	41	38	37
Number with information	132	194	135	466	142	159	503	184	229	131	334	68	31	101	29	69	319	63	53	Total 3342
Number without information	19	2	20	8	14	11	79	41	8	25	44	9	27	24	1	19	60	8	57	476

prior to hospitalization. In many cases, death is virtually instantaneous, but in others there is a significant delay between the onset of symptoms and death, which might be prevented by the more rapid institution of appropriate treatment. Death within the first few hours after infarction is frequently the consequence of arrhythmias which may themselves be fatal or may play an important role in the precipitation or aggravation of cardiac failure and shock. In most cases, arrhythmias can be treated successfully.

Although most deaths from acute myocardial infarction (AMI) occur outside hospital, the rate is also high (usually about 30%) in hospital in the absence of intensive coronary care. It is generally agreed that coronary care units contribute to a significant reduction in hospital mortality from AMI mainly because they permit the rapid detection and correction of arrhythmias. There is less information available about coronary care areas, which have been developed in many hospitals, but it would appear that a significant lowering of mortality may be achieved when they are appropriately equipped and staffed.

Mobile coronary care units have not been developed on the same scale as coronary care in hospitals. The extent to which they produce a further reduction in mortality has not yet been fully established. However, there is no doubt that they accelerate the administration of intensive care and may halve the time between the onset of symptoms and the availability of intensive care compared with the conventional admission system.

Intensive coronary care, as defined above, is only one of the phases in the management of the patient with AMI. These phases include the call for medical aid from the patient or an associate, initial treatment by a general practitioner or paramedical personnel, transfer to hospital by mobile coronary care unit or conventional ambulance, management in admission areas, transfer to and treatment in the CCU, subsequent care in a ward prior to discharge, and rehabilitation.

Care of the patient outside hospital

Because of the high mortality in the hours immediately following the onset of symptoms, the patient must receive skilled attention as soon as possible. The following recommendations are aimed at ensuring that he does so.

1. Members of the public should be informed about the symptoms of heart attacks and be made aware of the methods of summoning medical aid in emergencies.

2. Patients, particularly those with angina and previous myocardial infarction, and their close associates should be given professional advice about calling for aid without delay. Methods of obtaining emergency care for coronary patients should be made known to them.

3. General practitioners should be made aware of the need for a quick response to calls which suggest the possibility of AMI. A quick response means, in general, the immediate calling of an ambulance (mobile care) before trying

to reach the patient personally. They should be familiar with the operation of coronary care and mobile coronary care facilities in their area; furthermore, they should be trained in the diagnosis and management of AMI, especially cardiac arrest.

4. Staff of polyclinics and health centres should be trained in the management of cardiac emergencies, particularly cardiac arrest, and should be equipped with portable ECG monitoring apparatus and defibrillators.

5. In areas where the emergency ambulance service is staffed by doctors or by paramedical personnel fully trained in the management of cardiac emergencies, the ambulances should be equipped with monitors and defibrillators.

When general-purpose ambulances are used which do not have such highly trained personnel, it is necessary to ensure that all ambulance staff are trained in cardiac resuscitation. They should have available to them a means of obtaining help rapidly from those trained in the use of defibrillators and equipped with them.

The problems of intensive coronary care in areas with less than 100 000 inhabitants

Previous recommendations[a,b] have been largely concerned with the facilities which can be provided at major centres serving areas with populations of more than 250 000. For a variety of reasons, such recommendations may not be applicable to less populated areas. These reasons include the following:

(*a*) the relatively small number of cases in such areas may not justify the creation of a CCU in the nearest hospital;

(*b*) highly specialized medical, nursing and technical staff may not be available at all times; and

(*c*) patients may have to be transported over long distances.

There are great variations in these factors from one area to another. For example, in some areas with a low density of population, only a relatively brief journey is necessary to reach a major centre; in other areas, several hours' journey may separate the patient from even a low level of medical care. The appropriate form of treatment in these different areas will, therefore, depend on the distribution of population, the prevalence of ischaemic heart disease in the area and the general standards and availability of medical and nursing care.

---

[a] *The organization of coronary care units:* report on a Preparatory Meeting. Copenhagen, WHO Regional Office for Europe, 1969 (document EURO 5020).

[b] *The role of mobile coronary care units:* report on a Working Group. Copenhagen, WHO Regional Office for Europe, 1970 (document EURO 5020(2)).

Systems of care in areas of low population

Depending on the relationship of the rural area to a major centre and upon the transport facilities, the following alternatives are available:

(*a*) transport of patients to a centre with a CCU;

(*b*) the admission of patients to hospitals which have a coronary care area associated with an intensive care unit or medical ward;

(*c*) care in a hospital which does not have a coronary care area but can provide general nursing care and minimum resuscitation facilities; and

(*d*) care of the patient at home.

Transport of patients to centres with CCUs

This may be the best arrangement for areas of low population density not far from major centres, particularly if patients can be transported in conditions of intensive care. It is not thought that such a method is optimal when more prolonged journeys are involved, although it may be appropriate for the transport of specific patients (e.g., those with heart block requiring pacing) who may require further treatment in specialized centres.

Coronary care areas in hospitals which cannot provide a CCU

Intensive coronary care implies 24-hour medical cover. Coronary care areas can, therefore, only be maintained in hospitals which already have a service for acute medical and surgical emergencies. In hospitals which do not have enough patients with AMI to justify the creation of a CCU, the coronary care beds must be linked either to other intensive care facilities (preferably medical), if such exist, or to a medical ward. In either case, the general principles of coronary care design should be observed. The patients should be under close observation and be protected as far as possible by partitions or walls from the distressing and dramatic events which may occur in adjacent beds. When the coronary care area is included in an intensive care unit, it should form a distinctive part of it.

A physician who is fully trained in coronary care must be in charge of the area and be responsible for its administration, for the implementation of a protocol of procedures, and for staff training. He will require regular periods of retraining.

All medical staff who are concerned in the care of patients in the coronary care area must receive training in ECG interpretation, especially arrhythmia analysis, and in the management of the complications of myocardial infarction, including cardiac resuscitation. One member of the medical staff must always be readily available. As in coronary care units, the nurse-in-charge will be a key figure in the day-to-day care of patients and must have been fully trained in coronary care. Other nurses in the area should be trained in arrhythmia interpretation, in the management of myocardial infarction, and in cardiac resuscitation.

A coronary care area should be equipped with the following:

(*a*) ECG display oscilloscope with central ECG monitor with read-out system, heart rate display and alarms;

(*b*) oxygen and suction;

(*c*) signal system for obtaining help;

(*d*) defibrillators;

(*e*) resuscitation equipment;

(*f*) facilities for pacing the heart;

(*g*) equipment for intravenous infusions.

As technical assistance may be unobtainable, it is desirable that there should be spare oscilloscopes, ECG recording machines and at least one extra defibrillator. This should be in the form of a battery-operated portable defibrillator or a portable monitor-defibrillator.

It is important to ensure that all equipment, when installed, complies with a rigid safety code and that this code is observed in subsequent maintenance.

A therapeutic protocol which is appropriate for the particular unit is essential. This should include details of the admission and discharge criteria as well as instructions on the use of drugs for the prevention and treatment of arrhythmias, shock and cardiac failure.

In general, the therapeutic methods employed in coronary care areas will not differ from those in major centres. However, only in exceptional circumstances should electrical pacing be undertaken by a doctor who has not been fully trained in this in a major cardiac centre. (In those hospitals in which there is no such suitably trained individual available, it may be possible for a cardiologist to visit the hospital, insert a pacing electrode and then transfer the patient, if necessary, to a CCU under supervision.)

Care in small hospitals

In areas of low population density, with scattered communities, it is inevitably difficult to provide the type of coronary care defined above, which necessitates a 24-hour emergency service. Small hospitals should be strongly discouraged from creating "coronary care" facilities if continuous surveillance is not possible and if there is an insufficient number of cases to enable the doctors and nurses to gain sufficient experience or to maintain proficiency. However, even in such an environment, it is important that the staff should be trained in cardiac resuscitation, particularly as they may encounter cardiac arrest from a number of different causes such as anaesthesia, surgery, drowning and electrocution. Thus, they should be trained in cardiac resuscitation and in the use of a portable monitor-defibrillator. Furthermore, facilities should be available for the transport under intensive coronary care conditions of patients who require to be moved to a coronary care unit. For this purpose, transport by a coronary care ambulance, aircraft or helicopter may be necessary.

Care of the patient at home

In some areas and countries care in the home may not be possible, either for social or for medical reasons. However, it may be in certain situations unavoidable, or even preferable, that a patient should be treated in his home. The general practitioner must play an important role in the management of such patients by taking the responsibility as to whether they should be moved. In reaching this decision he must take into account the local circumstances, the social situation and the fact that a prolonged journey to a hospital which is not equipped for coronary care, particularly if some hours have elapsed after the onset of symptoms, may be medically inadvisable. The local doctor must also be responsible for the administration of analgesic drugs and, if necessary, oxygen and appropriate treatment for arrhythmias and cardiac failure.

Persons who live in isolated areas should, if possible, be instructed in dealing with medical emergencies and be provided with essential drugs for their treatment (as they are by the Flying Doctor Service in Australia). One individual in each community should be responsible for the supervision and administration of drugs. In such areas, it is highly desirable that advice by telephone or radio should be available quickly.

THE DEVELOPMENT OF CORONARY CARE
IN THE COMMUNITY[a]

The Working Group on the Development of Coronary Care in the Community, which was convened by WHO in cooperation with the Government of Belgium, brought together 16 temporary advisers from 10 Member States in the European Region and the USA.

The purpose of the meeting was to assess the relative effectiveness of treatment of patients with acute heart attack in coronary care units, general hospital wards and the home, to advise on the optimal length of hospitalization for such patients, and to make recommendations for improvement of continuous rehabilitation programmes.

It was expected that the conclusions of the Working Group would be of value in further development of community control of cardiovascular diseases and refinement of guidelines for the care of coronary patients in general.

To facilitate its discussions, the Working Group agreed on a number of definitions in respect of coronary care, which are listed below.

Definitions

Intensive coronary care is the continuous and intensive surveillance of patients suspected of having acute myocardial infarction (AMI), in order to prevent and treat its complications, especially arrhythmias. It may also comprise care of patients with other acute cardiac problems, including serious arrhythmias not due to coronary disease.

A coronary care unit (CCU) is a self-contained unit specifically designed for intensive coronary care.

A coronary care area is an area set aside for intensive coronary care, but not self-contained, and closely associated with an intensive care unit or a medical ward.

A mobile coronary care unit (MCCU) is a facility which enables personnel trained in coronary care to reach patients at the site of a heart attack (at home or elsewhere) as soon as possible, to start emergency treatment immediately, and to continue observation and treatment during transport to hospital.

---

[a] Extracted from: *The development of coronary care in the community:* report on a WHO Working Group. Copenhagen, WHO Regional Office for Europe, 1980 (document ICP/CVD 003(9)).

A mobile intensive care unit (MICU) is a facility which provides general or medical intensive care, including coronary care.

A community cardiopulmonary resuscitation (CPR) programme provides for resuscitation of patients outside hospital, training of the public in the principles and practice of CPR, and establishment of an MCCU or an MICU.

Comprehensive cardiac care refers to the systematic control of heart disease throughout its natural history. In the context of an acute heart attack, it comprises pre-hospital activities with community involvement, cardiac care in hospital whether in specific or general wards, and post-hospital care with emphasis on progressive rehabilitation and secondary prevention. Comprehensiveness and continuity are two essential characteristics.

Preliminary considerations

Overall mortality for patients after an acute coronary heart attack is in the region of 40% during the first four weeks; about 40% of the deaths during this period occur during the first hour, many of them instantaneously. There is good reason to suppose that many, if not most, of these early deaths are due to ventricular fibrillation in the absence of fresh myocardial necrosis (1). Patients with acute heart attacks, on the other hand, who survive the risks of the initial phase, have usually sustained a myocardial infarction and have symptoms which lead them or their associates to seek medical care, although after a variable period. It is these patients who are potential candidates for in-hospital coronary care. The risk of death in such patients is maximal during the first hour or so after the onset of symptoms and thereafter diminishes rapidly. Most of the early deaths are due to ventricular fibrillation occurring in the absence of evidence of severe disturbance of left ventricular function. In the succeeding hours, however, the risk of arrhythmic death becomes progressively less; when death occurs it is usually due to shock or heart failure or, less frequently, to rupture and thromboembolism.

During the early hours of AMI, when the risk is greatest, the symptoms may be unconventional, physical examination unhelpful and special tests often incapable of allowing a definite diagnosis. As a consequence, at the time when the decision must be made as to whether home or hospital treatment should be effected, it may be impossible to establish whether or not a myocardial infarction has occurred.

CCUs were created when it was appreciated that arrhythmias were a leading cause of death in patients presenting in hospital with the features of AMI and that such deaths could be prevented by appropriate interventions by skilled and properly equipped personnel. Subsequently, attention was turned to the use of therapy for the prevention of ventricular arrhythmias, to the management of atrioventricular block and other bradycardias and to the control of atrial arrhythmias. The most important aspect of the CCU was the congregation of patients at high risk under the supervision of skilled personnel using constant electrocardiographic monitoring and the appropriate apparatus for CPR. However, the concept that skilled nurses

74

should particularly devote themselves to the recognition of "warning arrhythmias" which precede ventricular fibrillation has been questioned as it has become apparent that the fibrillation may occur unannounced. Increasingly, one of two approaches is being employed in the prevention/management of ventricular fibrillation. In some units no prophylactic antiarrhythmic treatment is used but ventricular fibrillation is treated promptly when it occurs. In an increasing number of centres, however, it is becoming the practice to use lignocaine in a prophylactic manner in all patients with suspected myocardial infarction. However, careful administration with an infusion pump is necessary and the risks of toxicity have not been fully evaluated.

Although early experience suggested that measures to reduce the incidence of death from pump failure had been unsuccessful, current evidence indicates, but not conclusively, that in cases of disturbances of haemodynamic function adequate monitoring of pressures in the right and left side of the heart, early drug therapy, the support of respiratory function and the timely application of intra-aortic balloon pumping may help to decrease in-hospital mortality. Possibly, earlier surgical intervention in the appropriate circumstances will play an increasing part.

The CCU has also played an important role in most hospitals in the management of acute cardiac problems not due to coronary heart attacks. Thus, patients presenting with acute left- and right-sided heart failure, serious arrhythmias and conduction disturbances and shock are frequently cared for in the CCU environment. As such cases often form a substantial percentage of all those treated in a CCU, the term seems inappropriate; "cardiac intensive care unit" might be a preferable description.

In view of the expense and special skills which CCUs require, much attention has been paid to their cost-effectiveness. Rose (2), for example, has commented: "coronary care units are expensive consumers of scarce resources and it is unfortunate that there has been little attempt to evaluate their achievements". He also pointed to the failure of mortality from coronary heart disease to fall following the introduction of coronary care.

In the early days of CCUs consideration was given to the institution of randomized trials to test their efficacy, but it was not felt at the time that such trials were feasible. However, Hofvendahl (3) carried out a non-randomized trial comparing apparently similar groups of patients allocated to coronary care and conventional ward care on the basis of bed availability and claimed that there was substantially reduced mortality in the CCU. It was agreed, however, that there was not as yet conclusive evidence that the institution of CCUs reduces overall mortality significantly.

A WHO Working Group on the Organization of Coronary Care in the Community (4) commented that even if CCUs were effective it might not be possible to demonstrate an effect on community mortality from ischaemic heart disease (IHD) for the following reasons:

(a) sudden deaths which are not susceptible to treatment in a CCU form such a high proportion of deaths from IHD;

(b) the provision of CCUs has not been on a sufficient scale to meet the needs of the community; and (*c*) the facilities of CCUs have not been appropriately used, particularly with regard to the admission of patients at the earliest and most dangerous phase of an acute heart attack.

It is of interest that the mortality from coronary heart disease in the 35–64 years age group has been falling since 1967 in the USA, Australia and New Zealand where the institution of coronary care and mobile coronary care has been most rapidly promoted. The fall in the mortality in these countries cannot be attributed solely to the introduction of intensive coronary care but Reader (5) has calculated that such care may be responsible for 20–55% of the reduction.

Pre-hospital coronary care

It is now clearly established that many lives can be saved by the organization of pre-hospital coronary care. Initially, such care was provided in ambulances manned by physicians and usually initiated by patients reporting their symptoms to a general practitioner (6). Attention is now being concentrated on cases of sudden collapse in the community which may or may not be preceded by symptoms. Success in the resuscitation of these patients depends upon a comprehensive approach providing for education of the public in the principles of CPR and the availability within five minutes of rescue teams equipped with defibrillators. The effectiveness of this comprehensive approach has been demonstrated in Budapest and Seattle and other cities around the world. The institution of either of these components of the system without the other is undesirable and may be counterproductive.

In order to institute a pre-hospital care programme, training of the public in CPR and the organization of rescue teams must proceed *pari passu*. Patients, particularly those with angina and previous myocardial infarction, and their close associates should be given clear advice on how to call for aid without delay. Methods of obtaining emergency care for coronary patients should also be made known to the public in general.

All physicians, especially general practitioners, should be made aware of the need for a quick response to calls which suggest the possibility of an acute coronary heart attack. They should know how the mobile and other coronary care facilities operate in their area, and they should be trained in the diagnosis and management of myocardial infarction, especially cardiac arrest.

Although it has been shown that a mobile unit whose function is restricted to the care of cardiac cases may be valuable, it is felt that MICUs which deal with other forms of emergency are a more economic and effective means of bringing coronary care to the victim because of the possibility of providing them in large numbers and the difficulty of identifying the nature of the collapse shortly after its onset.

Although the ability to rescue individuals in the community has been amply demonstrated, the effect of such measures on overall mortality from IHD has not been established. Estimates of a 10–15% reduction have been made in Seattle but the coronary death rate in that community is not known. The Working Group considered that the development and assessment of CPR programmes in association with IHD registers should be strongly encouraged.

While community CPR programmes are the most effective way of preventing sudden, near instantaneous death, it is important that even when such programmes are not available, patients with suspected myocardial infarction should come under intensive care as soon as possible. Patients frequently delay calling for medical aid and the response of general practitioners is often slow. It is important for those responsible for coronary care in each community to consider how these delays could be reduced, whether by public or patient education, by the education of general practitioners, or by streamlining of the process of hospital admission.

Organization and functions of the coronary care unit

CCUs were introduced specifically to treat or prevent cardiac arrest in AMI, as described in extensive literature on the subject. In the 15 or so years since their creation, a more comprehensive approach to the management of patients with suspected or proven acute IHD has been developed and in fact different levels of care can be distinguished, as follows.

1. Facilities must be available for the evaluation of patients with suspected but not proven AMI. Many of these patients will eventually be shown to have a different diagnosis or to have sustained severe ischaemic pain in the absence of infarction. Others will have sustained a myocardial infarction and will be at risk from ventricular fibrillation in spite of the fact that proof of infarction is not evident. It is therefore important that the suspected infarction patients should be in an environment where the onset of cardiac arrest can be detected and treated immediately. While this may sometimes be done in an emergency department, it is more satisfactory for such patients to be assessed in an area within or adjacent to a CCU (7). Specifically designated "precoronary care" seems to be of value in particular local conditions.

2. Patients with definite but uncomplicated myocardial infarction require close observation within the first 24–48 hours because of the risk of serious arrhythmias and because they may develop complications. However, the nurse/patient ratio can be relatively low as long as the infarction is uncomplicated.

3. Patients who develop the more serious complications of myocardial infarction such as cardiac arrest, cardiac failure and shock require close observation and a high nurse/patient ratio. Artificial ventilation, haemodynamic monitoring or intra-aortic balloon pumping may also be necessary.

4. Similarly, patients with serious arrhythmias not due to myocardial infarction may require close supervision in the coronary care area. The CCU can be used to house all patients in categories 1–4, although it may be more economical to have two levels of coronary care: one with a high and the other with a low nurse/patient ratio.

5. Patients who have recovered from the acute phase of myocardial infarction remain at risk from cardiac arrhythmias in the succeeding days. These

patients and those with arrhythmias not associated with AMI are best cared for in an adjacent ward where monitoring, ambulatory ECG tape recording and perhaps telemetric facilities are available (a post-coronary or intermediate care area).

In some hospitals, particularly if they are small, it may be necessary to provide coronary care facilities on a more restricted scale as a part of a medical or general intensive care unit. Under these circumstances, the principles previously elaborated should still apply and the subunit should be under the direction of a physician with cardiological training.

It has been suggested that the need for CCUs in hospitals might be substantially reduced if home care was more widely accepted as a suitable form of management (see pp. 80–82). However, it is apparent from general experience and more specific studies in Bristol (*8,9*), Nottingham (*10*) and Teeside (*11,12*) that a substantial proportion of patients with myocardial infarction are considered to require treatment in hospital because of their medical condition or because of the social background. It is clear, therefore, that there is a need for specialized cardiac facilities in hospitals and that the decision to keep many patients at home would not materially diminish the demand for coronary care. It seems improbable that a more positive approach to home treatment would materially affect community costs in this regard.

Rehabilitation and duration of stay in hospital

In previous years, prolonged immobilization was considered necessary for the healing of a myocardial infarction. Recently, it has become evident that early mobilization does not usually impair cardiac function or subsequent prognosis, and permits a quicker return to normal activity. As a consequence, there has been a progressive decrease in the duration of bed rest and of hospitalization. While in general hospitals it is still widespread practice to retain uncomplicated cases for two or more weeks, in many leading cardiological centres the median duration of stay is now in the region of 10 days, the least complicated cases staying no more than 7 days. No evidence has been produced to suggest that such early hospital discharge is harmful but the optimum lengths of stay for different types of case have yet to be defined. It is clear, however, that the appropriate length of stay for a given patient must depend upon the prognosis, the effect of measures which might be expected to improve this, and upon social factors.

Prognostic indices (*13–18*) have proved valuable in deciding on the time of discharge from the CCU, the rate of mobilization during the early hospital phase, the length of hospital stay, and the likely benefit of secondary preventive measures during the post-hospital phase.

Several guidelines for mobilization are in current use. They are based essentially on the clinical status of the patient and the reaction to gradually increasing physical exertion (e.g., heart rate increase, chest pain and dyspnoea). The rate of mobilization varies markedly from one centre to another.

It can be said that the variables available at the bedside and in the early stage have good predictive power — probably as good as that of several complicated laboratory variables, which may not be available until later. It is also evident that, whatever indices are used, prognosis is largely dependent upon the extent of infarcted myocardium.

As stated, many institutions have found it possible to reduce the median stay of patients in hospital to 10 or 11 days without evident harm.

In the most favourable cases, hospitalization was restricted to one week. It is important to emphasize, nonetheless, that some patients require more prolonged care but that these can be largely identified on the basis of the prognostic indices referred to above.

Studies on factors influencing the prognosis for one to two years after AMI have been published in recent years. Age is a strong factor, as is the number of previous infarctions and the presence of left-sided heart failure as detected clinically and by other means during the acute phase. Other important factors indicating extensive myocardial damage include atrial fibrillation during the acute phase, high serum enzyme levels, persistent sinus tachycardia and cardiomegaly. Continuation of smoking after myocardial infarction seems to increase the risk of a future fatal event, even when the effects of other variables are taken into consideration. The same is true of the presence of hypertension before or after the infarction. The presence of hypercholesterolaemia has been associated by some with a poor prognosis, but in most studies it does not seem to have any influence.

With the aid of the variables mentioned it is possible to select groups with estimated mortalities ranging from 10–12% to about 80% during the succeeding five years.

The value of exercise tests in evaluating the prognosis of patients after myocardial infarction, including tests during the later period of hospitalization, are under active study. At present, no firm recommendations could be made on the value of such tests in the management of patients and further research is required.

Continuity of care

Continuity of medical care is of vital importance in the management of patients following an episode of AMI. Problems of continuity are frequently encountered in large hospitals even in regard to care within the hospital (emergency room, CCU or adjacent area, medical ward and outpatient clinic) because of the large number of physicians, nurses and other health personnel involved. They can be minimized if the patients are admitted directly to the CCU or adjacent area and, after spending the appropriate time there, are transferred to a progressive care ward under the supervision of the same group of personnel.

Continuity is often lost immediately after patients are discharged from hospital, which is particularly regrettable in the case of early discharge. Where general practitioners are involved in the further care of the patient, their precise responsibilities and those of the hospital must be clearly defined. At least one follow-up visit to the hospital is desirable and it should include both physical assessment and psychological reassurance. Differences of opinion and practice exist in regard to further follow-up. In some areas, a comprehensive rehabilitation programme is operated by the hospital clinic but in others it is left to the general practitioner to supervise the clinical care of the patient and the application of secondary preventive measures.

In hospitalized patients, it is essential that the different aspects of rehabilitation, including the amount of exercise to be undertaken and the prospects of returning to work, should be discussed with the patient as soon as possible after the acute phase is over. At this time the importance for the patient of stopping smoking, controlling weight, taking an appropriate diet and having adequate knowledge of the condition must be appreciated by the medical and nursing staff. The patient's relatives should also be informed about his capacities, the degree to which he should be cautioned or encouraged to undertake more, and the ways in which help may be obtained if further medical problems ensue. Written material should also be made available for the benefit of both the patient and his associates.

It is important that the comprehensive care programme should be organized by hospital physicians in consultation with the general practitioners of the area.

Home management

Because some general practitioners have claimed that the mortality of patients cared for at home was as low or lower than that reported by CCUs, it has been suggested that home care would be appropriate for some or even most patients with myocardial infarction.

To resolve this question, Mather and his colleagues in Bristol and the southwest of England carried out a trial, enlisting the help of a large number of family physicians spread over a wide geographic area who allocated patients on a random basis to home or hospital treatment (*8,9*). It was reported that there was no significant difference in mortality between those kept at home and those sent to hospital. Unfortunately, only 24% of the patients reported on were entered in the randomized trial, the remainder being electively admitted to hospital or left at home. The results of the trial were dismissed by a joint working party of the Royal College of Physicians and the British Cardiac Society on the grounds that "there were defects in its design, many patients were seen late after the onset of their symptoms and there was a small and ill-defined minority of the patients who were randomized".

Because of the uncertainty raised by the Bristol trial, it was felt necessary to conduct a randomized trial using a different basis for entry and allocation (*10*). In Nottingham a hospital-based team consisting of a junior physician and a CCU trained nurse was sent to patients' homes in response to calls from general practitioners about suspected cases of myocardial infarction. The team made an initial working diagnosis, provided emergency treatment, excluded unsuitable patients on predetermined grounds and observed the remainder of the patients in the home for a total of 2 hours. They then allocated them randomly to home or hospital management (26% of patients could not be randomized because medical or social factors determined hospital admission). Of 132 patients randomized to home treatment of suspected infarction, 13% died within 6 weeks, whereas 11% of 132 allocated to hospital treatment died within the same period. No statistical difference could be shown in the mortality of the two groups. It has been pointed out, however, that the team arrived at a relatively late time (median 3 hours) after the onset of symptoms and randomization did not occur until after about 5 hours. The numbers of patients studied were such that a clinically important result might not have been statistically demonstrable. Three patients survived to 6 weeks having been treated successfully for ventricular fibrillation during the period at home. There was significantly higher mortality in patients with myocardial infarction treated at home on the first day compared with those treated in hospital. Furthermore, 26 of those allocated to home treatment subsequently required hospital admission, chiefly because of the difficulty of relieving pain adequately at home.

A non-randomized comparison of home and hospital treatment was conducted in Teeside (*11,12*). This took the form of an observational study of all patients in a restricted geographical area, some of whom were kept electively at home and some of whom were sent to hospital, including a minority treated in a CCU. Mortality of 8.8% was observed in those kept at home, 12.9% in those treated in a CCU and 18.7% in those treated in general wards. Although the authors claimed comparability between those treated at home and in a CCU, the percentage of definite myocardial infarction patients was higher in the hospital groups than in those at home and the patients sent to hospital had requested and received medical care earlier than those kept at home. The authors concluded "this study is not intended to resolve the debate as to whether home or hospital is the best place to treat patients with acute myocardial infarction. It does indicate for those who have survived the 3-hour interval from apparent onset that the CCU may have little to offer".

The papers cited all suggest, some even in their title, that there is little to be gained by CCUs as opposed to home treatment. However, in all of the studies, those who were managed at home were seen at a relatively late period after the onset of symptoms and cannot be regarded as representative of all patients with AMI. It is wrong, in our opinion, to pose these opposites as a confrontation. Rather, both home and hospital treatment will have a place depending on the state of the patient and the time he is first seen. It is apparent from the natural history of this condition that intensive care for acute heart attacks can only make an impact on mortality if it is applied as early as possible. Home treatment can be instituted only if high quality domiciliary medical care is available. In many countries, neither the public nor the medical profession accept the concept of home care of infarction and hospital admission is invariable.

It is clear that home care has a place, in particular for those who are seen late after the presumed onset of symptoms and at that time appear stable. In contrast, hospitalization is indicated when patients have developed the major complications of myocardial infarction or when there are other diseases requiring hospitalization or when home support, either medical or social, is inadequate.

With regard to costs, it is evident that the greatest reduction in expense can be achieved by prompt and proper assessment of the risk of complications from AMI. The use of a multilevel intensive care unit in connexion with home care, when possible, offers the best solution. Furthermore, it should be borne in mind that such units with their varying nurse/patient ratio (ranging from 1 : 4 in pre-CCU care to 2 : 1 in the intensive care area with haemodynamic monitoring) must be organized in the framework of a community system providing for CPR and mobile coronary care in existing ambulance or fire-fighting units on the one hand and rehabilitation and after-care on the other.

Conclusions

1. Community-based CPR programmes are effective in preventing many deaths from acute heart attack. However, the effect of such programmes on the overall mortality from IHD has not been established because of the absence of IHD registers in the communities concerned.

2. Early ambulation and hospital discharge have been successfully instituted in many hospitals but not in others. While there is no evidence that the move towards earlier activity is harmful, definitive information on the optimal time for ambulation and discharge for different classes of patient has not yet been obtained.

3. While home care may have a place in the management of patients seen to be in good condition some hours after the onset of an acute heart attack, provided medical and social conditions are satisfactory, a high proportion of all those with heart attack will require hospitalization. The increased use of home care is unlikely to result in a substantial reduction in coronary care costs in the community.

4. The role of various interventions in the management of AMI is being actively investigated at present. Because of the uncertainty with regard to the value of such measures as routine prophylactic antiarrhythmic therapy, use of vasodilators, and intra-aortic balloon pumping, it is not thought that the *Manual on intensive coronary care* (*19*) could be satisfactorily revised in its present form. However, there is need for guidance of those developing coronary care facilities, which WHO should be in a position to provide.

5. Insufficient knowledge is available at present with regard to re-habilitation and secondary prevention. Further studies are needed to assess their value and the effectiveness of various methods of providing information on these subjects to the medical profession and the public. The work carried out by the International Society and Federation of Cardiology should shed further light on this matter.

Recommendations

1. The development of community CPR programmes should be encouraged in areas where they can be carefully evaluated. Simplified coronary heart disease registers should be instituted in association with intervention studies.

2. On the basis of existing information, early hospital discharge can be encouraged, although the optimal time in relation to the patient's condition has yet to be established.

3. There may be circumstances when home care is appropriate, e.g., when high quality domiciliary medical care is available for patients who are seen to be in good condition some hours after onset of the event or when a prolonged journey without intensive care might be hazardous. However, even when home care is available, hospitalization should be recommended for patients in the first few hours after the presumed onset of symptoms. In patients seen at a later stage, hospitalization is indicated for those who have developed major complications of infarction, those who have some other disease requiring specialized medical care, and those whose home support, either medical or social, is inadequate.

4. The *Manual on intensive coronary care* (*19*) should not be revised in its present form, but consideration should be given to the production of a booklet providing advice on the organization of coronary care.

5. Because of the need for progressive care and secondary preventive measures, continuity of care between the hospital and home must be ensured.

The Working Group agreed that WHO should encourage research in a number of areas as follows.

(*a*) Careful studies should be undertaken in areas with registers as to the effect of pre-hospital and hospital coronary care.

(*b*) Information should be collected which would permit determination of the optimal time of hospital discharge.

(*c*) Efforts should be made to develop means of determining whether specialized facilities during rehabilitation, such as clinics and sanatoria, make a contribution to the patients' rate of recovery.

(*d*) There is a need to implement previous recommendations that research be undertaken on the effects of community, patient and medical education on patient-induced and other causes of delay in hospitalization. Information which is currently available from both European and non-European sources should be collated.

(*e*) Further information should be obtained on the prognostic and therapeutic value of exercise testing programmes in rehabilitation after myocardial infarction.

(*f*) Further evaluation of secondary preventive measures, including drug treatment and surgery, should be promoted.

References

1. **Cobb, L.A.** et al. *Circulation,* **51**–52 (Suppl. III): 223–228 (1975).
2. **Rose, G.** *British journal of preventive and social medicine,* **29**: 147 (1975).
3. **Hofvendahl, S.** *Acta medica scandinavica,* **519** (Suppl.): 9–78 (1971).

4. *Organization of coronary care in the community:* report on a Working Group. Copenhagen, WHO Regional Office for Europe, 1976 (document ICP/CVD 003(7)).
5. **Reader, R.** *Circulation,* **58**: Part II, 32 (1978).
6. **Pantridge, J.F. & Geddes, J.S.** *Lancet,* **2**: 271 (1967).
7. **Hugenholtz, P.G. et al.** *Intensive care medicine,* **4**: 1 (1978).
8. **Mather, H.G. et al.** *British medical journal,* **3**: 334 (1971).
9. **Mather, H.G. et al.** *British medical journal,* **1**: 925 (1976).
10. **Hill, J.D. et al.** *Lancet,* **1**: 838 (1978).
11. **Colling, W.A. et al.** *British medical journal,* **2**: 1169 (1976).
12. **Dellipiani, A. et al.** *British heart journal,* **39**: 1172 (1977).
13. **Peel et al.** *British heart journal,* **24**: 745 (1962).
14. **Norris, et al.** *Lancet,* **1**: 274 (1969).
15. **Helmers, C.** *Acta medica scandinavica,* **555** (Suppl.) (1974).
16. **Moss, A. et al.** *Circulation,* **49**: 460 (1974).
17. **Vedin, A. et al.** *Acta medica scandinavica,* **198**: 353 (1975).
18. **Verdouw, P.D. et al.** *Circulation,* **52**: 413 (1978).
19. **Oliver, M.F. & Julian, D.G.** *Manual on intensive coronary care.* Copenhagen, WHO Regional Office for Europe, 1970.

THE LONG-TERM EFFECTS OF CORONARY BYPASS SURGERY[a]

Coronary heart disease is a major health problem and cause of death in Europe. Its manifestations are multiple and include sudden death, myocardial infarction, heart failure and angina pectoris. The last symptom occurs with varying degrees of severity. At its most extreme, patients are considerably handicapped and suffer from intractable pain. Although severe angina constitutes only a small fraction of the total problem, it has considerable implications for patient, doctor and society. Many patients will respond to medical management, but the development of coronary artery bypass grafting (CABG) has offered a new approach, especially for the severely handicapped.

The role and scope of coronary artery surgery in the treatment of CHD are not yet completely known. Clinical studies have suggested that considerable symptomatic improvement occurs in many patients, but discussion continues both in the USA and in Europe regarding the long-term effects of CABG on survival. Uncontrolled studies, especially in the USA, have raised the possibility of improved survival prospects for operated patients, but a simultaneous control group of medically treated patients has been lacking. Such controlled studies are now in progress in the USA and Europe, but only preliminary reports are available.

Controversy exists, not only because a surgical approach has become available but because the medical management of angina pectoris has advanced and may well improve the prognosis of patients with angina.

A Working Group on the Long-term Effects of Coronary Bypass Surgery was convened by the WHO Regional Office for Europe in The Hague from 1 to 4 November 1977. The purpose of the meeting was to review current evidence with regard to the indications and benefits of CABG, to assess the needs in Europe in this respect and to suggest what facilities were required. A final answer on the public health value of CABG was not expected from the Working Group.

The participants referred to recent advances in medical treatment and secondary prevention of coronary heart disease (CHD). Due attention was paid to the lack of knowledge concerning the areas of incidence and prevalence of angina pectoris in the community, and the need for further studies was stressed.

---

[a] Extracted from: *The long-term effects of coronary bypass surgery:* report on a Working Group. Copenhagen, WHO Regional Office for Europe, 1978 (document ICP/CVD 003(8)).

Possible influence of recent developments in drug treatment and secondary prevention on the natural history of coronary heart disease

The general picture of coronary heart disease is probably changing continually. This is suggested, for instance, by the fall in the death rate in the United States during the past 15 years.

There is increasing evidence, as yet not conclusive, that various medical measures improve the prognosis in patients with angina. Chief among these are the cessation of smoking and the use of β-adrenergic blocking drugs.

There is a strong correlation between cigarette smoking and death in patients with coronary heart disease. It has been shown that cessation of smoking after myocardial infarction is associated with a relatively improved prognosis. It seems likely that the prognosis in patients with angina, whether or not they have suffered infarction, would also be favourably affected by the cessation of smoking.

The overall cardiac mortality in patients with hypertension is favourably affected by antihypertensive treatment in that it prevents cerebrovascular accidents and cardiac failure. The failure by the Veterans Administration Cooperative Study Group on Antihypertensive Agents to show a reduction in coronary death rate does not disprove the possibility that more prolonged therapy would have had a more favourable result, or that other forms of antihypertensive therapy would have been more effective. Recent reports suggest that the treatment of hypertension with β-adrenergic blocking drugs may substantially reduce mortality from coronary disease.

Quite apart from their value in the treatment of hypertension, there is good reason to suppose that β-adrenoreceptor blocking agents may improve the prognosis in patients with coronary heart disease, even if their blood pressure is normal. Although this has not been proved in the case of angina, some studies indicate a substantially reduced mortality over 1–2 years among patients who take either alprenolol or practolol after infarction.

There have also been suggestions that anticoagulants, lipid-lowering agents and anti-platelet compounds improve prognosis, although the evidence on these measures remains debatable.

It is reasonable to assume that changes in medical management involving the above drugs or habits may also influence longevity after coronary surgery.

Clinical value and limitations of coronary bypass surgery

The objective of coronary bypass surgery is to obtain long-term optimal revascularization of ischaemic myocardium with minimal or no perioperative damage to the myocardium. Vessels eligible for grafting usually have at least a 50–70% reduction in lumen diameter and the number and length of stenoses have to be considered. The most widely used and tested bypass graft is that using an autogenous saphenous vein obtained from the leg, although other veins such as the cephalic vein of the arm can be used. The internal mammary artery has also been employed and is preferred in some centres. When the saphenous vein is used, one end is anastomosed to the aorta and the other to the affected coronary artery beyond the obstruction.

Multiple grafts can be inserted if necessary. When the internal mammary artery is used the dissected distal end of the vessel is grafted onto the coronary artery beyond the obstruction.

The Working Group reviewed the current knowledge concerning the risks and results of coronary bypass surgery. It emphasized that the proper evaluation of coronary bypass surgery will ultimately be dependent on the study of concurrent rather than retrospective control groups, since advances in medical therapy have taken place concomitantly with those of surgery.

Stable angina pectoris

Operative mortality has been steadily declining. In experienced centres coronary bypass procedures can be performed with an operative mortality of about 1–2% in low-risk patients with stable angina. The term "low-risk" is taken here to cover patients who are less than 70 years old, who have a normal-sized heart, good ventricular function (evaluated by left ventriculography), no recent myocardial infarction, no coexisting adverse medical diseases, and coronary arteries suitable for grafting. If one or more of these criteria are not met, surgical risk is increased. Other important factors increasing operative mortality are: left-main disease, diffuse coronary artery disease and substantially reduced ejection fraction of the left ventricle, especially below 0.3.

Perioperative morbidity has decreased with increasing surgical experience and improvement of parasurgical techniques. Today perioperative myocardial infarction clinically recognized by the appearance of new Q-waves occurs with a frequency of below 10%; the true incidence is probably higher. A further reduction can be expected in experienced centres. The short-term and long-term effects of perioperative infarction on cardiovascular function and prognosis are not well documented.

The incidence of pulmonary embolism is reduced if patients are routinely anticoagulated in the early postoperative period.

The main result of aortocoronary bypass surgery is improvement of angina pectoris in about 90% of the patients. In about two thirds of patients angina disappears completely. Clinical improvement, when combined with an improved exercise tolerance, is, in most instances, the direct result of revascularization. This can be demonstrated by postoperative evaluation of exercise tests, myocardial lactate metabolism and scintigraphic studies.

In patients with severe angina pectoris, the degree of symptomatic improvement and increase of exercise tolerance after successful surgery is usually far greater than can be observed with any other form of treatment available to date. This, in turn, directly improves quality of life and working capacity. The degree of symptomatic improvement declines with time, but for the majority of patients it lasts for years.

Symptomatic improvement is often sufficient to allow patients to return to work. However, a combination of social, economic and psychological factors may hamper optimal rehabilitation. The longer the period of inactivity before surgery, the less likely is a return to work. Once the decision has been made to operate, this should be done as soon as possible.

Improvement of ventricular function at rest — usually assessed by left ventriculography — has not been definitely demonstrated. Exercise or pacing-induced ischaemic conditions, such as pulmonary wedge pressure increase and segmental hypokinesia of the left ventricular wall, may at times improve following adequate revascularization. These haemodynamic studies during stress may become useful in evaluating the effect of revascularization on left ventricular function, although their value has not yet been completely substantiated.

The improvement or otherwise in symptoms and in exercise testing, including ECG, is generally related to the adequacy and completeness of revascularization as well as to possible subsequent graft failure. Vein graft patency rate is reported to be 80% or more after one year in most experienced centres; it may be higher when internal mammary arteries are used. After the first postoperative year the number of further graft occlusions is small; it is reckoned to average 2% annually. Factors influencing graft patency rate are surgical experience, appropriate patient selection, surgical technique, distal run-off, size of artery, site of anastomosis and possibly previous myocardial infarction in the area of the grafted artery. A number of surgeons believe that endarterectomy or jump grafts are possible methods of revascularization of totally occluded or distally stenosed arteries.

Reliable data on the effect of aortocoronary bypass surgery on the length of life are not yet available. Uncontrolled studies have shown that patients with multiple vessel disease may have improved survival following bypass surgery. This conclusion is not supported by the information available from controlled studies, a clear exception being patients with left-main disease. Significant improvement in survival has been shown for left-main disease in the Veterans Administration Cooperative Study with a small number of symptomatic patients. No data are available regarding asymptomatic persons with this lesion. The few randomized studies reported to date have demonstrated no differences in survival between operated and unoperated patients with other types of lesion, although a longer follow-up period may be required to evaluate the data fully.

The follow-up results are not as yet available from the two large controlled studies in progress: the European Coronary Surgery Study and the collaboration studies (CASS) sponsored by the US National Institute of Health.

No data are yet available for determining the effect of bypass surgery on the long-term incidence of myocardial infarction.

Unstable angina pectoris

The benefits of coronary bypass surgery in unstable angina pectoris are generally similar to those outlined above for patients with stable angina pectoris. Data available from the US Cooperative Control Study show no differences in mortality and rate of myocardial infarction between medically and surgically treated cases both during the inpatient period and after an average follow-up period of 24 months. Although many patients with unstable angina pectoris that is initially sufficiently severe to suggest acute myocardial infarction do develop a mild or even asymptomatic course after their discharge from hospital, there is a minority of such patients with unstable angina in whom intensive medical therapy may not control symptoms of recurrent ischaemia. Urgent operative procedures may be necessary under these conditions; operative mortality and postoperative infarction rate appear to be slightly higher, but the symptomatic improvement is essentially the same as in stable angina.

Life-threatening arrhythmias

Beneficial effects of aortocoronary bypass surgery on life-threatening arrhythmias (such as recurrent ventricular fibrillation and tachycardia) have been reported, but clear evidence is not available. There is a need for controlled studies.

Coronary artery obstructions in cardiac lesions for which surgery is indicated

Uncontrolled studies suggest that surgical mortality rates may be reduced in patients undergoing operation for cardiac conditions such as ventricular aneurysm, postinfarction mitral incompetence and aortic valvular disease, when coexisting stenosed coronary arteries are simultaneously grafted, even if angina pectoris is not present. Controlled studies are, however, very much needed.

Summary

Coronary bypass surgery improves the quality of life in the majority of properly selected patients, but there is no evidence, except for that provided by a small controlled study of patients with left-main disease, that it favourably influences longevity. The procedure is associated with mortality which has been reduced in low-risk patients. Perioperative complications have decreased although the true frequency and consequences of perioperative infarction have still to be established. Long-term postoperative follow-up of all patients is necessary because coronary bypass surgery is not a curative procedure for coronary arteriosclerosis. Appropriate medical management (correction of risk indicators, etc.) should continue after bypass surgery, since such measures may have a favourable influence on postoperative results.

Indications for coronary artery surgery

The Working Group was of the opinion that the available evidence regarding the advantages and disadvantages of CABG, as discussed in the previous section, requires that a distinction should be made between clearly established and less well established indications for revascularization. This distinction implies that surgery, according to less well established indications, should preferably be performed only at experienced centres where adequate evaluation of the results can be performed, so that these indications can be clearly established or discarded. It is thus recognized that the indications given below may change as new information becomes available.

Clearly established indications for bypass grafting

It is assumed that in all situations listed below a significant obstructive lesion is present as defined in the previous section.

1. Stable or unstable angina when there is an obstruction of 50% or more in the left main coronary artery.

2. Stable angina pectoris, sufficient to impair substantially the individual's usual level of activity, which has not responded to adequate medical treatment over a period of several months. "Adequate medical treatment" includes the correct use of the full therapeutic range of β-adrenergic blocking agents and other anti-anginal compounds, as well as treatment of conditions such as obesity, hypertension, anaemia and heart failure. In addition, the patient's lifestyle should be adjusted so that he has adequate physical exercise and rest and avoids sudden massive exertion and psychological stress. He should stop smoking.

3. Angina in patients with a cardiac lesion for which surgery is indicated.

4. Unstable angina pectoris:

(*a*) angina increasing in frequency, duration or severity, including pain at rest, and pain not responding to adequate medical therapy, and excluding acute myocardial infarction;

(*b*) recurrent episodes of unstable angina, as defined in (*a*).

Appropriate medical therapy of patients with unstable angina includes admission to hospital, bed rest, oxygen, adequate use of nitrates and β-adrenergic therapy, and other measures recommended under the treatment of stable angina.

Less clearly established indications

1. Patients without ischaemic chest pain but with a cardiac lesion for which surgery is indicated and in whom coexistent coronary narrowing has been shown by angiography. Such conditions include:

(*a*) sequelae of myocardial infarction: ventricular aneurysm, post-infarction ventricular septal defect, mitral incompetence due to rupture of papillary muscle or chordae tendineae;

(*b*) valvular, especially aortic, heart disease; and

(*c*) congenital heart disease.

2. Cardiogenic shock due to left ventricular failure without surgically remediable mechanical abnormalities.

3. Mild angina pectoris in patients with multiple vessel coronary artery disease.

4. Asymptomatic persons with stenosis of more than 50% of the left main coronary artery.

5. Diffuse distal atherosclerotic disease.

Contraindications to operation

Certain conditions exist in which the risk involved in an operation may outweigh the potential benefits and thus may be considered contraindications to operation. These include:

(*a*) acute myocardial infarction;

(*b*) cardiac failure due to diffuse myocardial scarring and without ischaemic pain; and

(*c*) associated terminal diseases or chronic diseases that will affect longevity.

Methods and procedure of patient selection

The Working Group realized that important changes are occurring in the recognition and treatment of coronary heart disease. Thus it is only possible to supply guidelines rather than clearcut indications for investigative methods and procedure.

Methods

1. History and physical examination are the most essential parts of the evaluation of the patient being considered for CABG. Great care should be taken to assess the disability due to angina pectoris since this is the major indication for or against coronary arteriography and CABG in most patients.

2. Other laboratory investigations. Routine laboratory tests, ECG at rest, chest X-ray and haemodynamic studies provide information which may be important in evaluating contraindications for surgery or in assessing the results of operation rather than in defining indications for coronary arteriography and CABG.

Additional studies are currently under assessment and these may become useful in the evaluation of myocardial ischaemia and left ventricular function.

3. Exercise ECG test. A markedly positive exercise test — ischaemic ST-depression of more than 2 mm and/or abnormal heart rate and/or pathological blood pressure response — is considered to suggest serious coronary artery disease such as main stem or multiple vessel lesions in symptomatic patients and, therefore, strongly reinforces the indication for coronary arteriography.

The risk of serious complications is very low and does not limit the use of the exercise ECG test to any appreciable degree. The most important limitation of the test is the considerable variability of its sensitivity and specificity in indicating anatomical lesions. This variability depends on the type of test, the patient's symptoms, the resting ECG and complicating conditions and treatment. Nevertheless, an adequately performed test is useful even if its diagnostic value is limited, because it helps to evaluate individual physical capacity and to assess the effect of any treatment on this capacity.

4. Coronary arteriography. There are no absolute means for identifying a patient suitable for CABG short of coronary arteriography and left ventriculography and, therefore, selection of candidates for this investigation may present considerable problems, at least as far as certain groups of patients are concerned. The investigation is not free of complications. The risk of fatality is 0.1–0.3% while the risk of myocardial infarction is about 3–5 times higher. The hazard of angiography is increased in individuals with main stem disease. Particularly distressing, however, is the fact that there is considerable variation in the evaluation of "surgically significant" coronary artery lesions. Factors involved include the lack of quantified techniques for evaluating the degree of obstruction, observer fatigue, surgical bias on the part of the observer, poor quality of the film, and psychological factors. Films that cannot be interpreted owing to an incomplete investigation should be regarded as an important complication. In general, the more experienced the centre, the lower the complication rate.

Indications for coronary arteriography

It is understood that contraindications to CABG will have been excluded when indications for coronary arteriography are being considered.

1. Severe stable angina pectoris as defined above.

2. Serious suspicion of left-main disease. Left-main disease has been found in 3–11% of patients with arteriographically demonstrated coronary disease. Only in less than 1% is the obstruction isolated. Association with multiple vessel disease is an important feature. Although the history may indicate varying degrees of pain, a high proportion of patients with a main left stem lesion have accelerating, severe or unstable angina. Another important feature is that these patients frequently exhibit a markedly positive exercise ECG test quite independent of the severity of angina.

Most patients with a main stem lesion will be detected if coronary arteriography is performed on the following indications:

(*a*) evaluation of patients with severe, stable or unstable angina as previously defined;

(*b*) evaluation of patients with markedly positive exercise test as previously defined.

While the broad use of exercise testing for identification of candidates for coronary arteriography can be considered in patients with mild angina, it is not recommended in asymptomatic persons. The likelihood of a false positive test is too high and the number of normal arteriograms obtained would be unacceptable. For persons in certain occupations, e.g. airline pilots, an annual exercise testing may be performed routinely. In these situations an exercise test must be markedly positive to warrant coronary arteriography in the further evaluation of the asymptomatic subject.

3. Unstable angina pectoris, defined as chest pain which is increasing in frequency, duration or severity, including pain at rest. Coronary arteriography should be considered indicated only after all adequate therapeutic measures to control the pain have been attempted. Evidence should be present that significant myocardial infarction has not occurred.

4. Coronary heart disease without angina pectoris. Coronary arteriography is indicated in the following situations:

(*a*) preoperative evaluation of patients with a cardiac disease, especially aortic valve disease, for which open heart surgery is being planned; the result of coronary arteriography can provide better myocardial protection during surgery;

(*b*) after resuscitation from ventricular fibrillation of unexplained origin; in such cases patients will usually have rather severe multi-vessel disease, sometimes including left main stem lesion;

(*c*) patients with a markedly positive exercise test as previously defined.

Coronary artery surgery needs, attitudes and resources

Evaluation of the CABG needs in the community should be based on the prevalence and incidence of angina pectoris which meets the criteria for surgery set out above. There does not appear to be adequate information available on the prevalence and incidence of angina pectoris in many communities. It is emphasized that this assessment is based on currently available data. The conclusions are necessarily tentative and may well require subsequent revision.

Prevalence studies

These have assessed the prevalence of angina pectoris mainly by the use of self-administered questionnaires. Their clinical validity is not proven, although it is believed to be reasonable. Samples of prevalence rates of angina pectoris available include:

England — questionnaire (Rose, 1964): 3.6% of males aged 35–64 years;

Scotland — questionnaire (Lorimer et al., 1974): 5% of males aged 40–65 years;

Europe — WHO Prevalence Study — Rose questionnaire: 3.5% of males aged 40–59 years;

WHO European Multifactor Preventive Trial — Rose questionnaire: 4.4% of males aged 40–59 years.

Some data are available on the prevalence of angina in a typical British general practice:

Total no. of subjects:	2500
No. of patients with angina:	20
No. of patients with hypertension:	25
No. of patients with heart failure:	30

Prevalence of angina extrapolated from these data: 0.8% of this population.

Incidence studies

The annual incidence of angina pectoris in the community has been assessed from various studies:

Health Insurance Plan (New York, 1969):	0.22% in middle-aged males;
New Angina Study (Edinburgh, 1972):	$\approx 0.2\%$ of males aged 30–64 years;
Seven Countries Study (Europe):	0.28% of males aged 40–59 years.

Since males aged 30–64 years represent approximately 20% of the population, this implies that, in a total population of 1 million, 400 males aged 30–64 years will develop angina each year.

In addition, angina will develop in a significant number of those over 65 years old and in a smaller number of female subjects. Angina is, however, a variable symptom and up to 50% of those experiencing pain will experience it only temporarily.[a] The number who develop angina for the first time and in whom it persists will be augmented by those in whom angina, apparently quiescent, has returned and in a proportion of those who have survived a myocardial infarction but have developed angina.

Annual number of patients requiring surgery

The following table is based on data relevant to countries which have an incidence of angina comparable to selected areas of Europe. It is assumed that approximately 10% of subjects with angina will have symptoms sufficiently severe to warrant operation. This assumption is based more on consensus of opinion than on hard data. The number is higher for those with post-infarct angina.

---

[a] The following results were obtained in a study (Seven Countries Study) of patients with angina pectoris (AP) on entry. After five years 37% had no AP; in 30% AP was still present; 13% had MI or worse CHD manifestations; 13% had died from CHD, and 7% had died from other causes.

	New angina	Post-infarct angina
Total with angina	*400*	*100*
Warranting operation	40	25
Incremental from previous years	40	–
Angina not sufficient to dictate surgery, but left main lesion present	20	–
Annual cases requiring surgery	100	25

Thus 125 new male cases would develop each year per million population. The proportion of females developing angina is smaller — perhaps 20% — a figure consistent with the typical fraction of current surgical cases. The total number of new patients meriting surgery for relief of severe angina is thus approximately 150 per annum per million population.

Backlog of patients requiring surgery

It should be noted that the above tentative figures refer to the incidence of new cases requiring surgery. There is a backlog of patients in the community with significant angina.

Current prevalence of angina:	0.8% = 8000 per million
Proportion of cases in 65+ age group:	50%
No. of cases less than 65 years old:	4000 per million
Proportion of cases of severe angina:	10%
No. of cases requiring surgery:	400 per million

Total need of coronary surgery in the community

The estimate for CABG need would be a backlog of 400 patients per million with the addition each year of 150 new patients per million for a country with incidence and prevalence rates similar to those cited. These rates will vary from country to country.

Depending on the rate at which the backlog is dealt with, the initial demand should gradually reduce over the years to a stable level unless the indications for surgery are altered. Long-term planning should take these factors into account.

Factors exist which may tend to increase the indications for surgery, e.g., proven saving of life, improved operation results and increased incidence of coronary heart disease. However, factors may also act in the opposite direction, e.g., improvements in the non-surgical management of coronary heart disease and decreased incidence of coronary heart disease. For purposes of current planning these possible tendencies are probably of less significance than the errors of estimate of the basic figures of current incidence and prevalence of disease and the fraction of these patients meeting the criteria for surgery listed above.

Demands for coronary surgery

The demands for surgery depend on a number of factors.

1. *Attitude of physicians.* Physicians' belief in the efficacy or otherwise of surgery for angina pectoris is an important factor. Thus, the San Francisco Bay Area Study reported at the meeting by Hultgren is of interest. Projections for coronary artery surgery needs in 1980 were made, based on whether the referring physicians had a "conservative" or "aggressive" attitude to surgery. A conservative physician is defined as a doctor referring patients for surgery only for relief of angina that does not respond to medical treatment. An aggressive physician is one referring patients for surgery on the basis of a significant obstructive lesion on the coronary angiogram. If all physicians were conservative the needs for surgery would be 230 per million population, while if all were aggressive the needs would be 1000 per million.

2. *Patients' attitudes.* These are affected not only by the opinion of the physician but also by information obtained from friends, other patients and the mass media. The level of disability that is accepted as tolerable is also important and is likely to vary from community to community.

3. *Resources.* In Europe at present the limited resources for coronary artery surgery have restrained demand. On the other hand, it must be recognized that in some countries the over-provision of facilities (both investigative and operative) may lead to exaggerated demands for investigation and surgery in order to justify the investment.

Resources and financial implications

The cost of coronary artery investigation and surgery provided by several centres in Europe was estimated at around $10 000 per patient, within a range of $5000–$15 000 per patient. The higher figure is likely if the projected optimal surgical facilities outlined above are used. However, any cost assessment must take into account not only the immediate cost of one regime but also the long-term cost of management of a patient by one regime in contrast to another. Thus, the probable higher annual cost of long-term medical management has to be considered.

In making a cost–benefit analysis, benefits are much more difficult to quantify in monetary terms. However, before any judgement can be made that coronary artery bypass surgery is expensive or inexpensive, comparable analyses are required of other medical and surgical therapies that are widely accepted, as well as alternative forms of therapy and prevention of CHD and their effectiveness.

96

From the patients' point of view, the relief of pain is the main benefit. In many cases this will permit the return to work of those who would otherwise be unemployed. Successful re-employment depends not only on successful surgery but also on local economic and social factors such as trade union regulations, employers' attitudes, the level of unemployment and social legislation.

Conclusions

1. Up-to-date data on the prevalence and incidence rates of angina in different countries are required, as are facts related to the degree of disability and the social consequences of this.

2. The pool of patients requiring coronary artery surgery according to the criteria set out in this report represents both a backlog of patients of about 400 per million population and an annual incidence of new patients of about 150 per million population. These figures refer to a country with a prevalance and incidence of angina similar to certain areas of Europe already studied, and will have to be considered for each area separately: in some the need will be greater, but in most of them it will be less.

3. These conclusions are tentative and may require revision in the light of further epidemiological information or alterations in the critiera for surgery.

Guidelines for optimal resources for coronary bypass surgery

In formulating guidelines for the planning of optimal resources for coronary artery surgery, the Working Group took into consideration a number of recommendations from several published reports as well as the experience gained in certain European centres. The Group considered it essential that the envisaged centre should provide for other surgical procedures, such as operations for valvular disease, congenital cardiac disorders and possibly vascular surgery.

The maintenance of optimal standards

In order to maintain high standards of quality care for patients undergoing open cardiac operations, an optimum number of 12–15 operations per week should be performed in each centre. The optimum-sized centre should therefore provide for approximately 500–550 open heart operations per year. Smaller centres with an annual capacity of 250–500 operations might be considered under special circumstances.

The cardiac surgical team

It is stressed that the cardiac surgical team can only work efficiently when integrated with the medical cardiology team. The available services should therefore provide comprehensive cardiac care on a 24-hour basis.

The centre for 500–550 operations per year should be staffed by 4 staff surgeons, supported by 10 junior medical staff who should preferably include trainees in cardiovascular surgery at different stages.

Approximately 50 coronary bypass operations are required per year per surgeon for adequate professional skill to be maintained.

The anaesthetic team

This should include 4 staff anaesthetists supported by 3 junior medical staff. These services should be designed to provide 24-hour cover to the operating room, the intensive care unit and, if necessary, the catheter laboratory.

Technical staff for perfusion and monitoring

The ideal number of perfusionists for the envisaged cardiac surgical centre of the size defined above is thought to be 4. In addition, 3 physiological measurement technicians are required. There should be adequate arrangements for the maintenance and servicing of equipment.

Theatre

Three theatres are considered to be necessary for this workload. This takes into consideration the necessity for emergency operations and the need to provide a potential for an expanding workload.

Beds

Thirty-eight beds, of which 6–8 are equipped and staffed for intensive care, are required. In addition, facilities for combined intensive care and isolation should be provided.

Perfusion and monitoring equipment

Four pump oxygenators and 2 intra-aortic balloon counterpulsation units are necessary. Adequate monitoring equipment should be available in all 3 theatres and all intensive care beds.

Nursing staff

Twenty-two nurses, of whom 12 should be qualified, are required to staff the 3 theatres. In the intensive care unit, 30 nurses, of whom 25 should be qualified, are required (4.2 nurses per bed). For the ward, 25 nurses, of whom 15 should be qualified, are required.

Blood transfusion and pathology laboratory facilities

Facilities for clinical biochemistry, microbiology and blood transfusion and physiotherapy should be available 24 hours a day.

Cardiac medical and radiology team

While it is not the primary purpose of this report to consider the resources for cardiac medical services, it is stressed that the cardiac medical component is considered to be an integral part of the envisaged centre. This should include 4–5 cardiologists supported by 4 junior medical staff, 2 assigned to angio rooms (catheter laboratories), and 4–5 radiographers.

Availability of other medical disciplines

The centre should have adequate links with other medical disciplines, particularly renal dialysis units.

Staff for documentation of results

Two secretaries should be provided for documenting results of operations, including follow-up data.

Summary and conclusions

Coronary heart disease will remain a major burden to the community in the coming decades. Severe angina is a relatively rare manifestation of the disease, but it presents a dramatic clinical picture which can in many instances be alleviated by surgery. In one small study a significant improvement in survival rates has been shown in patients with left-main disease. There are no reliable data showing differences in survival between operated and unoperated patients in other categories.

Coronary bypass surgery should be seriously considered in the following situations:

(*a*) severe stable angina not responding to optimum medical therapy;

(*b*) unstable angina not responding to optimum medical therapy;

(*c*) symptomatic left main coronary artery disease.

There may be further indications, but these are less well established and are under continued investigation. Centres beginning coronary surgery should confine themselves to established indications.

Preventive and curative measures likely to ease the burden of CHD should continue to be sought and applied. Needs for coronary surgery in each community will vary according to the prevalence and incidence of CHD and the clinical load of the defined categories which should be established for each area. Examples of calculation of need based on specific prevalence and incidence rates of angina pectoris have been presented.

The optimal facilities for surgery have been presented. The centres should be large, capable of performing 500–550 operations per year. They should be closely affiliated with a larger medical community.

Possible areas of further research

Further data need to be accumulated concerning the prevalence and incidence of angina in each community.

More objective evidence of degrees of disability and severity of pain is required.

Continued studies are needed on the course and effect of surgical intervention. Standardized protocols are desirable.

Research in centres of excellence should continue to assess the importance of left-main disease and multiple vessel disease in asymptomatic patients.

Ways of identifying patients prone to sudden death should be studied further.

COMPREHENSIVE CARDIOVASCULAR CONTROL PROGRAMMES IN THE COMMUNITY[a]

Z. Pisa & T. Strasser
Cardiovascular Diseases
World Health Organization, Geneva

Cardiovascular diseases are, in all countries where reliable statistics exist, an important cause of death (*1*). In industrialized countries, nearly half of total mortality, one third of permanent invalidity, and 10–20% of patients' visits to "first-line doctors" are due to these diseases (*2*).

While at present cardiovascular diseases are only of public health importance in some parts of the world, there are definite signs that in future this problem will become worldwide. The control of infectious diseases and the increasing standard of living, with improving health care, are leading to an increase in the middle and old age groups. By the year 2000, life expectancy should range from 70 to 80 years of age in the industrialized countries, and from 60 to 65 years in the developing world (*3*). This will result in an increased frequency of chronic diseases, and specifically cardiovascular diseases.

One of the important tasks facing the medical profession today is, therefore, not only to control cardiovascular diseases in countries where they are highly prevalent but also to influence the countries which are undergoing industrialization; when reaching a higher level of development, these countries should not face the same problems as the developed world does now.

The amount of knowledge accumulated by cardiovascular research since the Second World War is voluminous; its application in general practice is, however, largely unsatisfactory. Cardiovascular diseases have not received the public health attention they deserve.

The importance of these diseases in many parts of the world requires a community approach in addition to care for the individual patient. The present situation could be improved by proper application of existing knowledge about the control of cardiovascular diseases in the community health services.

Terms of reference

The suggested *approach* is a community cardiovascular control programme integrated with the existing system of organization of medical care delivery as established in the respective areas or countries.

---

[a] Taken from Annex XXIII to: *Comprehensive cardiovascular community control programmes:* report of a WHO Meeting. Geneva, World Health Organization, 1975 (document CVD/76).

The *aims* of a cardiovascular disease control programme are to prevent disease, to reduce mortality and morbidity, and to help cardiovascular patients return to as normal a place as possible in the life of the community.

A "community" in this context means a group of people living in a defined geographical area.

The term "control" refers to measures related to all aspects of health promotion and protection.

Elements of a control programme include:

— prevention

— detection and early diagnosis

— treatment, including rehabilitation

— education of health personnel as well as the public

— research

— evaluation of activities and results achieved.

A certain level of organization of medical care is a prerequisite.

The reason for using the existing organization of medical care is the extent of the problem of cardiovascular disease in the community and the high frequency of other diseases in the middle-aged and old-aged population from which most of the cardiovascular patients are recruited.

Possibilities for control resulting from present knowledge

Hypertension. Hypertension is the most prevalent cardiovascular disturbance in virtually all parts of the world.

While there is uncertainty about the systematic treatment of symptomless persons with mild elevation of blood pressure, the treatment of severe hypertension is an important public health problem. The medical profession should be made fully aware of it. Measurement of blood pressure should become a part of every medical examination.

Nationwide screening programmes for high blood pressure are, on the contrary, not recommended. The reasons are that, on the one side, the impact of such measures has not yet been assessed, and, on the other, such action could unnecessarily overload the health services. Because of lack of knowledge in this respect, wherever possible, such programmes could be started and experiences very carefully collected and evaluated on a pilot basis.

A WHO cooperative study on programmes for the control of hypertension at the community level is now being carried out in 15 centres in all WHO regions (*4*). It was confirmed that half of the persons who have elevated blood pressure are not aware of it, half of those who are aware of it are not treated, and of those treated, only half are treated properly and their blood pressure controlled. The project covers a total of approximately 800 000 people. It includes screening, registration and follow-up of the patients, education of physicians in the community, and health education of the public. The project is expected to finish in 1979–80. It will show the difference between a systematic control programme for hypertensive patients compared to the existing care as applied in different communities, and also the influence of control of blood pressure on the incidence of complications, specifically in the groups of patients with moderate elevation of blood pressure.

Ischaemic heart disease. In spite of the great interest in prevention and control of ischaemic heart disease among populations of industrialized countries, the final effect on mortality and morbidity of all recommended measures is still limited.

The significance of risk factors has repeatedly been discussed (2) and there have been many intervention trials trying to influence the incidence of ischaemic heart disease. The problem of primary prevention of coronary heart disease as approached today, rests on the lack of definite evidence that, by introducing preventive measures in the middle-aged population, we can influence the incidence of atherosclerotic complications.

More and more, the tendency is to link the required changes in behaviour (nutrition, change in smoking habits, control of hypertension, improvement of physical fitness, control of diabetes, improvement of the environment) with a healthy style of living rather than directly with the prevention of cardiovascular diseases. It is therefore quite natural that new hope is given to the studies of precursors of atherosclerosis in children. The purpose is to intervene in the first or second decades of life in order to prevent the development of risk factors, rather than to try and change the risk factors in the middle-aged person when the atherosclerotic process is already advanced.

While patients could and should be advised by their doctors as to how to change their risk factors, if detected, mass screening programmes on a nation-wide scale are not yet recommended.

In the field of medical care for patients with coronary heart disease, great advances have been made. However, in spite of the development of intensive coronary care, its impact on mortality in the community is very limited.

WHO's myocardial infarction register project (5) has shown that among those under the age of 65 years, approximately 40% who suffer a heart attack die during the first 4 weeks; 33% of these die during the first 30 minutes after the onset of symptoms, and nearly half of this mortality occurs during the first 3 hours. Considering the delay in calling the doctor, which is on average one hour, any sophisticated intervention has only limited effects.

The problems related to the care of patients, together with rehabilitation of patients after myocardial infarction, are very well covered elsewhere (2,6).

The basic problems in the control of ischaemic heart disease are primary prevention as the most effective means of influencing the natural history of the disease in the community, the identification of persons at risk of dying suddenly or of having myocardial infarction, and assessing the effect of systematic rehabilitative and secondary preventive programmes in patients after myocardial infarction. All these questions are also being studied by WHO (6,7). Further laboratory research on the pathogenesis of atherosclerosis is also needed.

Stroke. There is evidence that age-adjusted mortality figures for cerebrovascular accidents are decreasing in several countries.

A certain number of stroke cases could be prevented if the blood pressure in hypertensive patients could be properly controlled.

A WHO cooperative study (4) has now collected information on more than 6500 cases of stroke. The annual incidence of stroke varied among different centres from 1.3 to 3.2 per 1000 inhabitants and the incidence rate, as expected, increased sharply with age. About half of the patients had hypertension prior to stroke. Only about 60% of those with hypertension had been treated. About a quarter of the patients died within one week and one third died within three weeks. Of those patients who had been comatose at onset 80% died, compared to only 15% of those who had been fully conscious. Past history of stroke, acute myocardial infarction, hypertension and diabetes did not appear to have much influence on the prognosis. One third of the surviving patients were able to resume some work after three months, but more than half required assistance in daily activities.

From the point of view of the community, control of high blood pressure is of particular importance. Cerebral infarction, like ischaemic heart disease, is closely associated with atherosclerosis. The measures designed to prevent atherosclerosis in connexion with coronary heart disease are therefore also relevant to the control of stroke in the community. Early diagnosis is also of paramount importance. Patients with transient ischaemic attacks should therefore be brought urgently into contact with doctors, preferably neurologists, who should decide about their further treatment.

Properly equipped and staffed hospitals should have a sufficient number of beds available for stroke patients in the acute phase. It is necessary to assess the indications for emergency treatment and to plan the subsequent rehabilitation, including secondary prevention. These facilities can be arranged within the framework of existing hospital services without implying the establishment of special stroke intensive care units; the value of these has not yet been proved.

It has also been shown that the long-term treatment of stroke patients and rehabilitation procedures do not necessarily require highly specialized rehabilitation units. Stroke patients under 70 years of age are often rehabilitated in general medical wards. Due attention has to be given to early activation and physiotherapy. An important part of rehabilitation is speech therapy. The psychological effects of communication with neighbours is of utmost importance and influences the whole development and cooperation of the patient. A very big obstacle to improving care is the negative approach of the medical profession in some communities.

Further research is needed in diagnosis to differentiate ischaemia and haemorrhage specifically. Marquardsen (8) further reports that, in his recent autopsy study, it was found that 4% of deaths considered to be of cerebrovascular origin were due to tumours, abcesses or some other cause.

Chronic chest diseases and cor pulmonale. Knowledge of the prevalence of this problem in the community is very limited. Surprisingly enough, the etiology is also not satisfactorily elucidated. The problem is underestimated in most communities. Recent surveys on patterns of mortality from respiratory diseases in different European countries suggest that etiological factors, such as infections and smoking, operate at different stages of life and that their relative importance varies from country to country (2). Public action against smoking, air pollution and industrial dust might be quite important in this respect. After the Clean Air Act of 1956 in the United Kingdom there was a decrease in mortality due to bronchitis in Greater London, as well as in industrialized parts of the country (2). However, the major factor of individual pollution, namely smoking, is not easily influenced. Other etiological factors of chronic diseases are advserse social conditions and hereditary factors.

Giving up smoking is of utmost importance in patients with early bronchitis.

Vigorous treatment should be introduced in repeated respiratory infections in children. These infections may form the first stage of chronic lung disease. The long-term consequences of such experiences in childhood are evident at the age of 21 when it is possible to detect the cumulative effect of early chest disease and current smoking habits on frequency of productive cough and other symptoms of early chronic lung disease (9).

It is possible to expect that, by influencing the progress of chronic bronchitis with bronchial obstruction, bronchial asthma and emphysema and, in some countries, also pneumoconiosis, a certain effect will be achieved in respect of prevention of cor pulmonale.

In spite of the fact that development of chronic chest diseases can be affected by currently available treatment, it is not yet recommended that mass population screening be introduced. However detection, registration and long-term follow up of patients predisposed to asthma or to respiratory infections should be introduced.

Rheumatic heart disease. The effectiveness of penicillin has been proven both in the prevention of first attacks (primary prevention) and of recurrences (secondary prevention) (*10,11*). Benzathine penicillin given intramuscularly is clearly superior to penicillin given in tablet form; its efficacy in preventing relapses is estimated to be seven times greater than that of tablets (*12,13*).

It is estimated that, to prevent 100 cases of rheumatic fever, it is necessary to treat 200 000 cases of acute sore throat (*14*).

The recommendations of WHO for secondary prevention, i.e. for prevention of recurrences of rheumatic fever and of deterioration of rheumatic heart disease, are described in detail elsewhere (*11*).

Pilot studies on the control of rheumatic heart disease in the community are now being conducted by WHO in 10 population centres in the Regions of Africa, the Americas, the Eastern Mediterranean and South-East Asia. The Organization assists with streptococcus studies in Egypt to promote the prevention of rheumatic fever. Furthermore, the project includes a study on the assessment of diagnostic critiera.

Considerable efforts on the part of the patient, family, school teachers and health workers are required to carry out such a programme.

The preliminary assessment of the results of WHO studies confirms the decisive role that social and economic factors play in the effectiveness of the control programme.

Present experience shows that the best results are obtained in areas where socioeconomic measures are coupled with a medical approach.

Congenital cardiac malformations. Knowledge of the etiology of congenital cardiac malformations, the prevalence of which is approximately 1% among live-born infants, is very limited. It is stated that chromosomal aberrations and hereditary syndromes account for approximately 5% of all cases (2). These malformations, like others, are common in rubella and thalidomide embryopathy. The implication of virus infections in the etiology is suspected. This uncertainty results in the fact that if any prevention can be done, rubella infection of the mother in early pregnancy should be avoided. It is also stated that pregnant women should avoid drug consumption and radiation, especially during the first trimester of pregnancy.

It is important that the symptoms and signs of congenital cardiac malformations are recognized very early after birth. Surgical treatment should be carried out in centres with great experience, since the results of the surgery will be much more beneficial.

Because of the high incidence among the newborn, special attention should be devoted towards educating physicians, nurses and other medical personnel to be able to deal with the problem as well as with related social and family aspects.

In planning services and care for the patients it is necessary to consider the psychological aspects of the child and the family.

The whole area needs extensive stimulation of research, especially as far as etiology and pathogenesis are concerned. The different therapeutic and surgical procedures should be evaluated, not only concerning mortality, but also regarding the functional results.

Organization of control programmes

As mentioned earlier, in establishing the community cardiovascular control programme, the existing system of organization of medical care delivery in the area or country should preferably be used. After a trial period, the new control programme should be integrated into the existing system.

As the organization of the services differs in different parts of the world, even in different areas, it would be very difficult to develop a uniform model. It is therefore recommended, at this stage of development, to establish a programme adapted to the specific conditions and health care system in a well defined population area on an experimental basis. Data should be collected and processed in order to evaluate continuously the impact of the measures introduced. This information would facilitate further planning and development. The costs of the programme and the need for resources should also be monitored. All this information would help the public health authorities in their future planning to eventually extend the programme.

Plan of operation for a community control programme

Considering all the details, a plan of operation must be prepared in advance. It should include and deal with objectives and goals, area of operation, methods and strategy, actions and measures to be taken, models of implementation, evaluation procedures, information system to be used, plan of training and education activities and, eventually, suggestions for research directly connected with the implementation of the programme.

Registers have proved to be of extreme value for the collection of information and data.

In its previous activities WHO has prepared and tested protocols for establishing registers for patients with acute myocardial infarction (*5,15*), for persons with elevated blood pressure (*4*), stroke (*4*), and rheumatic heart disease (*16*).

A register is, in principle, a pool for standardized recording and observation of the development of an acute or suspected case of a cardiovascular disease. It requires that a permanent record be established, that the case be followed up, and that the basic statistical tabulations be prepared both on frequency and survival, eventually for other purposes.

The register can only justify its existence if it can provide information which will be useful for the planning and evaluation of the service. As long as the data are collected only for registering the number of cases, the value is very limited and the efforts invested are not justified.

The WHO myocardial infarction registers have already been used and have proved their value in studies on primary and secondary prevention, evaluation of mobile coronary care units, evaluation of the effects of rehabilitation, and studies of prodromal symptoms of myocardial infarction.

As the registers record all the cases that occur in an area, the information can also be used as a tool for assessing the epidemiological situation for different cardiovascular diseases and trends that can occur. They have, furthermore, contributed to the improvement of the quality of care for patients, and through the information they provide, increased the attention of the public health authorities to the problem of cardiovascular diseases in the community.

Proposal for a comprehensive control programme in a community

Design of the programme

The programme consists of a coherent system of prevention and care, covering the total population in the area, together with an information system; it is based mainly on the existing health services which, however, may need to be restructured to some extent and complemented with preventive services, depending on the local situation.

The programme and its information system are focused on the individual, not on the disease.

As mentioned, particular emphasis is put on prevention.

Coherence. The term "coherent system" implies that the many facets of prevention and care are closely linked; that there is a constant exchange of information between general practitioners, specialists and, if pertinent, hospitals; that there is a community-wide plan of health education, equally pervading, say, general practice and hospitals; and that uniform diagnostic and therapeutic criteria are applied at all levels of health care.

The information system. This is the backbone of the programme. It collates information from all levels by registration procedures and acts as a tool both for following up registered individuals and for monitoring trends in the community. It is the instrument for carrying out surveillance and for evaluating the effect of the programme.

Use of available health services. As a matter of principle, the existing health services are used as much as possible. Establishment of new cardiovascular superstructures for the special purpose of the community programme is out of the question. Most solutions to the problems are within the competence of existing general health services, some of them within the competence of existing polyclinics and hospitals. Establishment of a body (board, committee, centre or institute) dedicated to the programme may facilitate the carrying out of the project. In areas where the existing organization of the services does not meet the requirements for ensuring the success of the programme, the existing services and facilities will have to be restructured, and will have to be complemented with the missing components, e.g. educational and epidemiological activities.

Record linkage. To preserve unity of the programme, information will be focused on the individual himself, rather than on his disease. This means that any data pertaining to an individual will be linked, e.g. the same individual will not be registered separately as a hypertensive patient, a subject rehabilitated after a myocardial infarct, and a person with a high risk.

Approaches

The key approaches of community control of cardiovascular diseases are: continuing education of health personnel, followed by intensified health education of the public and improvement of health services, searching for disease and for the risk of disease. All of these approaches are planned simultaneously. The relative intensity of each of them depends on local factors and will be determined according to the detailed analysis of the local situation.

Continuing education of health personnel has several facets. It encompasses both physicians and other health personnel. Within these crude groups, several levels are distinguished, such as continuing education of general practitioners and internists. The principal objective of continuing education is introduction or reinforcement of knowledge of prevention of cardiovascular diseases and striving to achieve motivation for preventive activities — at present a weak point in medical education.

Health education of the general public may become a pivotal component of the comprehensive community programme. There are two crude groups of health educational undertakings: education of patients (or high-risk people) and members of their family; and education of the healthy population, at various levels and ages.

The objective of health education is to change people's behaviour in order to make them actively participate in the cardiovascular control programme. If thoughtfully applied, health education may motivate receptive members of the public to such an extent that the public itself starts exerting pressure on the medical profession to increase preventive activities, contributing in this way to physician motivation. A detailed programme of health education should be worked out on the basis of an analysis of the actual situation.

Adjustment of health services and health care delivery should be based on an analysis of the actual situation in the community. Data on this subject may be available or should be made available by special purpose surveys or investigations.

An example of the possible approaches to improving health services is given by the ischaemic heart disease registration study, where analysis of the delay in hospitalization of infarct patients shows various reasons in various communities. The emergency care for ischaemic heart disease patients can thus be improved by taking special, goal-directed measures, such as providing a special telephone number for emergency calls, improving gate-to-ward procedures in the hospital, etc.

Many other examples for improving services could be given. This part of the programme also needs to be carefully elaborated, based on a preparatory study of the local situation.

Screening is based on the concept that early diagnosis may have a powerful secondary prevention value. Search for risk situations may have an even more important bearing on primary prevention of the major cardiovascular diseases. Both approaches should be combined in screening programmes.

Screening can be done in two ways: casually or systematically.

Casual (incidental) screening means that physicians are requested to use any contact with their patients to examine them for cardiovascular diseases or cardiovascular risk factors. Thus, for instance, blood pressure should be measured as part of any medical examination, or serum cholesterol may be determined when a blood sample is drawn, say for ESR. A significant part of the population sees a physician each year, therefore the yield of casual screening may be quite considerable.

Systematic screening is a special additional undertaking. Whether systematic screening is justified should be assessed locally. If the decision to organize systematic screening has been taken, the rate of screening should be established according to the capacity of the services to provide care for the detected cases, including counselling and follow-up examinations for identified high-risk people. It should follow present time-schedules. The plan must not have the character of a campaign, but should become a continuing, regular activity. It should be built into the plan of work of the general health services, which might be assisted by mobile screening teams, if judged necessary. A three- or five-year plan should be elaborated in this respect, covering within this period the various enterprises or other population groups to be screened. The scheme should be revolving, starting anew in the next period.

Operations research is an important, later-stage component of the comprehensive community control programme. Surveillance of the trends of morbidity, mortality, disability, indices of health services utilization, of effectiveness and efficiency of health measures, response rates to health education, etc., is providing valuable information which should be fed back to the programme and should be used for modifying the programme whenever desirable. Periodic evaluation of the effects of the comprehensive community control programme is a necessity. This evaluation will be carried out once a year.

Preparatory work

A series of preparatory substudies needs to be carried out. These substudies should produce the elements necessary for the planning of the approaches outlined above. The approaches will eventually be formulated as subprogrammes.

Demographic data. Basic demographic data and vital statistics are needed on the community, as follows:

- age and sex structure of the population
- mortality rates: general mortality and breakdown according to major ICD categories
- trends of mortality
- projections (if available) for the next two decades
- population morbidity (stability) indices.

A description of the demographic characteristics should be complemented by a map of the community indicating, if possible, population density in various parts of the territory.

Preparatory study of epidemiological situation. This study consists of a review of available data on the prevalence and incidence of cardiovascular diseases in the community. As it is very likely that available data are limited, it seems advisable to start at the same time a cardiovascular survey of a representative (random) sample of the population. This survey should produce data on present underdiagnosis and overdiagnosis of cardiovascular diseases, and on underutilization and possible overutilization of health services.

The epidemiological survey should be complemented by a possible simple exploratory assessment of knowledge, attitudes and practices in the population concerning cardiovascular diseases; this exploration should produce a basis for planning the subprogramme for health education.

The final product of this preparatory study should be a comprehensive "community diagnosis" of the present situation in the community, with respect both to the occurrence of cardiovascular diseases and to the existing control measures. Though of no bearing on the *concept,* the data are indispensable for defining the priority targets for action and planning the details of the comprehensive control programme.

Survey of available data. The following data are of interest:

- incidence of sudden death (forensic data)

110

- incidence of myocardial infarction and stroke (hospital data)
- number and percentage of hospital admissions and of days spent in hospital for cardiovascular diseases
- number of outpatient visits for cardiovascular diseases and structure according to diagnoses (if available)
- number of prescriptions for and cost of cardiovascular drugs (if available)
- number of emergency calls for cardiovascular diseases (true and "false" alarms)

These data will serve both for planning the project and for monitoring future trends when it comes to evaluating the effects of the programme.

Population sample to be surveyed. The sample to be screened should be representative and chosen at random. The population-based data thus obtained will serve as a measure of the "baseline" or pre-programme situation. Survey of a 3% sample of the total population is suggested. The sample should be drawn at random from the total population. Any of the acknowledged methods of drawing the sample may be used, but the use of random number tables is preferred. A target response rate of 95% is envisaged. Nonresponders must be followed up.

Examination of the surveyed persons includes: identification; age and sex; height and weight; blood pressure; ECG; serum cholesterol; simple personal history; simple history of awareness of disease (if any); diagnosis.

Cardiovascular patients, identified on screening, will be put on the community register in the next phase of the programme.

Preparatory study of resources. Resources should be carefully assessed in advance, in order to make the project viable. Study should be made of:

- health manpower of various categories
- facilities for cardiovascular care, their structure and capacities
- health educational resources
- managerial manpower and resources
- resources for data processing
- finances.

Particular attention should be paid to computer facilities, capacities for processing punch-cards, and available knowledge in data processing and analysis. An estimate of the volume of information should be made and it should be critically assessed whether the prospects for a smooth run of the project are realistic.

While an analysis of the epidemiological situation will produce a formulation of the *needs,* a summary of the resources will state the *constraints* of the eventual comprehensive control programme. An inadequate organizational set-up may put another constraint on such a programme. The final programme will have to be a compromise between the needs and constraints.

Registration and the information centre

Purpose of registration. All subjects diagnosed as having any cardio-vascular disease — ischaemic heart disease, stroke, hypertension or other — as well as sudden deaths, are registered on a special data form. The task of the information centre is to carry out cardiovascular surveillance in the community, i.e. to:

— monitor morbidity, mortality, and different trends in health care in the community; and

— assure follow-up of diagnosed patients by sending out enquiries if no follow-up has been reported to the information centre.

To make registration practicable, only a few selected, simple data will be recorded.

Data to be registered. A draft proforma of the suggested record form is given opposite. It contains all data to be registered. They can be put on a single punch-card. The registration form itself can be replaced by a punch-card.

Diagnostic criteria. The diagnostic criteria for myocardial infarction, stroke and hypertension are contained in early WHO documents *(4,5)*. They will be extracted and eventually presented in a separate booklet which will be used both as an appendix to the project manual and as a teaching aid in the subprogramme of continuing education of health personnel.

Operation of the information centre. The input to the information centre is the data outlined above. These data are recorded by all physicians on the special record form and sent to the information centre at regular intervals. The information centre itself or the commissioned electronic data processing centre transfers the data without delay to the electronic data file. Automatically, a search is made by computer for possible previous registration of the subject and, if confirmed, the new record is linked with the previous one. Record linkage is based on the identity number and checked by comparing sex and date of birth.

Periodically, the information centre makes automated searches for follow-up records that are overdue. In the case of a missing follow-up record, the computer automatically prints a letter to the patient, inviting him to pay a follow-up visit to the physician.

Hospital admissions and discharges, sick leaves, retirement and death are also reported to the information centre.

Redundant registration should be discouraged. However, it is safer to err by taking too many records at frequent intervals than by not following up the registered persons at the correct time.

Once a year the information centre produces a report containing an analysis of the cardiovascular situation in the community, with special reference to disease incidence, mortality, working incapacity, drop-out rates, health services utilization, etc. One of the main purposes of the information centre is to provide continuing surveillance of the cardiovascular situation in the community.

Registration ☐☐

Family name . . . .   First name . . . .

Year of birth ☐☐☐☐   Sex ☐☐   Identity number ☐☐☐☐☐☐☐☐☐☐

Date: Day ☐☐   Month ☐☐   Year ☐☐☐☐

Event: (enter X only in one single box)

Outpatient examination	☐	Home visit	☐	Retired due to disease	☐
Radiological examination	☐	Hospital discharge	☐	Death	☐
Hospital admission	☐	Sick leave started	☐	Other	☐
		Sick leave finished	☐		

Cardiological diagnosis: *Other diseases:*

Hypertension	☐	Cor pulmonale	☐	Diabetes	☐
Myocardial infarction	☐	Rheumatic heart disease	☐	Kidney disease	☐
Angina pectoris	☐	Heart failure	☐	Other	☐
Stroke	☐	Other heart disease	☐		
No organic heart disease	☐				

References

1. *World health statistics report,* **27**: 563–652 (1974).
2. *The prevention and control of major cardiovascular diseases:* report on a Conference. Copenhagen, WHO Regional Office for Europe, 1974 (document EURO 8214).
3. *World health statistics report,* **27**: 670–705 (1974).
4. *Community control programmes for stroke and hypertension:* report on a Working Group. Geneva, World Health Organization, 1971 (documents CVD/71.3 & CVD/72.1).
5. *Ischaemic heart disease registers:* report on the Fifth Working Group. Copenhagen, WHO Regional Office for Europe, 1971 (document EURO 8201(5)).
6. *Evaluation of comprehensive rehabilitative and preventive programmes for patients after acute myocardial infarction:* report on two Working Groups. Copenhagen, WHO Regional Office for Europe, 1973 (document EURO 8206(8)).
7. *The prodromal symptoms of myocardial infarction and sudden death:* report on a Working Group. Copenhagen, WHO Regional Office for Europe, 1971 (document EURO 8203(3)).
8. **Marquardsen, J.** *The natural history of acute cerebrovascular diseases.* Copenhagen, Munksgaard, 1969.
9. **Colley, J.R.T. & Brasser, L.J.** *Chronic respiratory diseases in children in relation to air pollution:* report on a study. Copenhagen, WHO Regional Office for Europe, 1980 (EURO Reports and Studies, No. 28).
10. WHO Technical Report Series, No. 126, 1957 (*Prevention of rheumatic fever:* Second report of the Expert Committee on Rheumatic Diseases).
11. WHO Technical Report Series, No. 342, 1966 (*Prevention of rheumatic fever:* report on a WHO Expert Committee).
12. **Feinstein, A.R.** et al. *Journal of the American Medical Association,* **206**: 565 (1968).
13. **Spagnuolo, M.** et al. *New England journal of medicine,* **285**: 641 (1971).
14. **Strasser, T.** Il controllo della febbre reumatica [The control of rheumatic fever]. *La clinica terapeutica,* **59**: 15–28 (1971).
15. *A simplified registration system and continued surveillance of ischaemic heart disease:* report on a Working Group. Copenhagen, WHO Regional Office for Europe, 1974 (document EURO 8201(7)).
16. *WHO programme on rheumatic fever prevention:* report of a Consultation. Geneva, World Health Organization, 1972 (document CVD/72.2).

STUDY OF THE PRECURSORS OF ATHEROSCLEROSIS[a]

Introduction and basic design

General aims

The need to detect precursors of atherosclerosis and to study prevention of the disease in childhood was recognized by a group of WHO consultants who met in Geneva in February 1974, and was emphatically reaffirmed at a second WHO consultation in October 1977. The purpose of the collaborative study described in the present protocol is to activate a study in accordance with the recommendations made at the consultations. The study to be carried out has two basic components: a cross-sectional survey among children[b] and adolescents of school age (6–15 years) and of their parents, and an optional longitudinal extension of the observations among all or a sample of the children.

Two fundamental questions require answers. One question is related to the distribution among children of the risk factors which are recognized as predictors of diseases due to atherosclerosis in adults. Are there differences in distribution already at an early age between parts of the world where such disorders are common and those where they are less frequent? The other question is concerned with identifying at an early age those children who are likely to be predisposed to becoming adults with elevated risk factor levels, in order to institute preventive measures at a time when they can be presumed to have the greatest chance of success. The proposed research project is intended to provide some answers to these questions and set the stage for further inquiry into methods of prevention and the determinants of geographic and individual variations.

The main risk factors chosen for these studies are serum cholesterol and blood pressure. It is also desirable to measure serum triglycerides and glucose tolerance. They are included in the common protocol as optional items. They require obtaining blood specimens in the fasting state but, from the experience of several studies carried out in schools, this requirement

---

[a] Taken from the appendix to the report of the WHO/ISFC Meeting on Precursors of Atherosclerosis in Children, Geneva, 1977 (document CVD/78.1).

[b] The important early years before the age of six — when dietary modification might best be introduced — are omitted at this stage of the study for practical reasons.

115

does not present a major logistical problem. Records on smoking will be obtained for older children and adolescents and obesity will be assessed. Family history and the presence of risk factors or disease in parents will be considered in relation to risk factors in children.

Cross-sectional survey

The cross-sectional survey constitutes the backbone of the collaborative investigation. It provides data on the distribution and age-trends of risk factors in children, permits geographic and sociocultural comparisons and serves as the basis for family studies and prospective investigations.

Children are approached through the school rather than the family because of easier accessibility and the possibility of carrying out more representative sampling. For reasons of economy, it is proposed to limit the age groups (both sexes) to 6, 9, 12 and 15 years. While sampling of all ages would be optimal, such grouping will serve immediate needs. If each centre recruits 100 children in each of the five age groups, the total of 400 constitutes a manageable load. These numbers are *minimal* since they must be analysed separately for boys and girls, even though current information suggests that sex differences in risk factors at a young age are absent or small. They may be augmented if feasible.

Attention must be paid to choosing groups of children who can be described in terms of the sociocultural environment to which they belong. This may be relatively easy in places which are rather homogeneous in this respect, such as some cities or rural areas. In towns where children from different socioeconomic environments attend different schools it may be best to select, say, three schools characteristic of three socioeconomically definable sections of the community and to examine 30–40 children in each school from each of the five age groups. It will be most practical to examine entire classes.

Clearly, the sampling must be adapted to local conditions. In case of doubt, WHO should be consulted for discussion of any problems. It is important to choose children in a way which permits their characterization in terms of their social environment, in order to be able to interpret any differences between studies. This is more valuable and practical than attempting the task, usually impossible with small numbers, of sampling children truly representative of a large region.

The matter of family studies and reasons for doing them are discussed in the report of the 1974 WHO consultation. In brief, family surveys obviate in part the need for long-term cohort studies because they permit a tentative estimate of whether a child is likely to belong to a high-risk group. For the immediate purpose of the present collaborative investigations, it is thought adequate to examine only the parents of the children, though participating groups are free to add other first-degree relatives. The examination of parents is optional but considered highly desirable. The inclusion of parents, of course, triples the number of examinations and calls for the establishment of special examination schedules. However, the effort is expected to be well justified in terms of the supplemental yield.

116

In order to interpret fully the findings on risk factor distributions within and between studies, knowledge of regionally customary and individual eating habits is necessary. Nutrition surveys belong to the field of the nutrition specialist, experienced in field surveys. There is no easy way of doing this type of investigation. It is therefore suggested that cooperating centres contact a local nutrition specialist or institute, discuss with a competent person which method to choose, and ensure continuous cooperation of the specialist and of his team for the duration of the study.

The choice of method will depend to a considerable extent on practical considerations, such as previous experience of the nutrition specialist with a particular method, financial and manpower resources, availability of locally validated food tables, and local habits and other sociocultural characteristics. Three groups of methods may be considered for use: the 24-hour or 48-hour recall method, the family consumption method, and the weighing method. The last one is considerably more expensive and elaborate than the recall or consumption methods, and the additional benefit may not always warrant its use in the context of the present study.

Knowledge of habits and their cultural and individual determinants is basic to their modification for the purpose of introducing preventive measures. There are, at present, no readily available instruments to serve these purposes. As the studies progress, collaborators should work together towards developing suitable questionnaires.

Longitudinal studies

The proposed longitudinal extension of the cross-sectional studies covers a period of three years. It is optional but highly desirable. While yearly re-examination of the cohort defined by the cross-sectional baseline survey is optional, a second examination at the end of three years serves the immediate needs. Taking into account the constraints of technical and short-term biological variation, the re-survey will permit identification of the children who show more marked risk factor changes with age than others, and the relating of such changes to the level in the parents, in an effort to characterize the group of children most likely to belong to a high-risk group later in life.

The cohorts of children and adolescents aged 6, 9, 12 and 15 at the baseline survey will be re-examined three years later. The same inquiries will be made and measurements[a] carried out as at the initial survey. If, in the interim, new ideas for research have developed, based on analysis of the baseline data or from other sources, these may be incorporated in the second survey. Also, if there is reason to suspect that risk factor levels in the population as a whole have changed, a new group of 9-, 12-, 15- and 18-year-olds may be compared with previously examined children who have now reached these ages and with their levels three years earlier.

---

[a] Comparison with initial values has to take into account random variations resulting in "regression to the mean".

117

For the comparison of risk factor trends in time among children with risk factor levels (and possible evidence of cardiovascular disease) among their parents, it is desirable to re-examine the parents too, for a second measurement will improve the accuracy of assigning a parent to a given risk category. If, as envisaged, a prevention study will also be done, the second survey will also serve as the starting point for such investigations.

Prevention study

The prevention study will be family-based. This type of preventive programme constitutes a new and needed approach since ongoing trials are essentially designed for individuals at high risk. Families for the prevention study will be chosen on the basis of the level of risk, as defined by single or multiple risk factor elevations in one or more family members. A preventive programme will be initiated among the families of children from one school, with another school supplying comparison families.

The effect of these programmes will be assessed by the reduction of risk factor levels in the family as a whole. Detailed guidelines remain to be prepared. There is little experience at present with such intervention studies. The methods of intervention, however, should suit the sociocultural characteristics of the population and therefore may not be uniform. A diversity of approaches has not only a greater likelihood of success but provides a means of comparing the success of different methods in various settings.

It is apparent that such investigations are the logical extension of the observational studies among children and their parents, and that it is hardly acceptable to limit research on atherosclerosis precursors solely to descriptive studies. These should be conceived as a first stage, eventually to be followed by the intervention study.

Pathology of atherosclerosis in childhood

The need for further knowledge on the geographical distribution of atherosclerotic lesions during the first two decades of life was stressed in the report of the 1974 WHO consultation. The collection of autopsy material in the areas where the examinations of schoolchildren are carried out would have many advantages, among others the comparison between prevalent risk factor levels and the extent of lesions. As the field studies are getting established, procedures for pathological studies should be developed.

Protocol of survey

Adherence to the present protocol and standardization of methods is a fundamental requirement for comparability of local studies.

Sources

The present protocol is based on the report of a WHO Consultation on Adult Cardiovascular Diseases in Childhood, in Geneva in 1974, and on the discussions and amendments proposed at the Second Meeting on Atherosclerosis Precursors, held in Geneva in 1977. It largely makes use of the methods applied in the Westland Schoolchildren Survey, 1973, described by Uppal et al. (Annex IV of the 1974 report). Further sources include: G. Rose & H. Blackburn, *Cardiovascular survey methods,* Geneva, WHO, 1969; J.M. Tanner, *Growth at adolescence,* Oxford, Blackwell, 1962; S.X. Uppal, *Coronary heart disease: risk pattern in Dutch youth,* Thesis, Leiden, 1974; WHO Technical Report Series, No. 231; and M. Long et al., Blood pressure recording in children, *Archives of disease in childhood,* **46**: 636 (1971).

Objectives

The general goal of the study is to produce information on possibilities and methods of primary prevention of coronary, cerebrovascular and other forms of atherosclerosis by promoting health in childhood and adolescence.

The collaborative field studies proposed are, of necessity, limited to the distribution and determinants of risk factors and studies aimed at their reduction. Intervention trials aimed at testing whether control of risk factors in youth will actually reduce disease would require (short of methods to measure lesions *in vivo*) decades of observation among many thousands of participants and cannot be realized at present.

Under more specific objectives of the study, answers to the following questions are expected.

1. What is the distribution of risk factors of coronary atherosclerosis as they originate or present in children in different environments?

2. How do they relate to risk factors in their parents?

3. How do they relate to disease in their parents and, possibly, grandparents?

4. When and in what circumstances do the risk factors appear and how do they evolve?

5. What differences can be detected in children between findings in areas of various adult morbidity rates and in various sociocultural settings?

6. What should be done to modify the risk factors as early as possible?

7. To what extent is intervention effective to prevent the development of high-risk factors or reduce them if present? (It is understood that the presence of risk factors is not synonymous with atherosclerosis.)

The first, second and third questions may be answered by cross-sectional study; question four implies longitudinal investigation; question five involves cross-sectional and multi-centre study, and questions six and seven include intervention.

Approaches

Groups of children living in defined communities (or territories) will be studied, if possible together with their parents.

Firstly, a cross-sectional study is made as a basic minimum and extended longitudinally wherever possible. This involves examination of the children (answer 1); history-taking of their parents (answer 2); and, optionally, also examination of the parents (answer 3). School-age children, of 6, 9, 12 and 15 years, are included; the inclusion of younger children — with different methods of examination — may be considered at a later stage.

Secondly, whenever possible, a longitudinal study will be made. Children and adolescents in the sixth, ninth, twelfth and fifteenth year are re-examined each year for three years or, if this is not possible, after three years only. Thus, an "assembled" longitudinal study from 6 to 18 years of age is obtained within three years, as a replacement of a true longitudinal study (answer 4).

Approaches to intervention studies and appropriate methods may be elaborated at a later stage.

Groups to be studied

Four age groups are investigated: 6, 9, 12 and 15 years. An age group includes subjects born in a calendar year, regardless of the month and day of birth. A minimum of 100 children and adolescents is enrolled from each age group — equal numbers of girls and boys. Preferably, whole classes are selected. Older or younger children belonging to the same classes may also be examined, but only those belonging to the specific age groups are counted and included in the eventual analysis. Either one primary school and one high school are selected, judged by the investigator to be typical for the area, or two (at most three) of them are chosen from socioeconomically contrasting areas of the community. Whenever possible, both parents are included in the study.

Exclusions, if any, from participation or analysis should be stated.

Procedures for organizing the survey

No rules can be given on how to organize the survey locally. Investigators have to observe local conditions. The procedures described in the report of the Westland Study may serve as an example in a given social environment.

Some general guidelines are as follows.

Cooperation with school authorities and school health services must be secured. Parents and children must be informed of the aims and methods of the study well in advance. Consent of the parents (or guardian) must be obtained.

Efforts should be made to have the parents examined as well. In places where this is not possible, however, history-taking by questionnaire may be accepted. The questionnaires may be taken to the parents by the children, as was done in the Westland Study. Even if the parents are

120

examined, the questionnaire may be handed out for completion in advance in order to gain time, but should be checked by a trained interviewer (nurse or clerk) when the parents appear for examination.

Glucose tolerance and triglyceride examinations are optional; if carried out, they require previous fasting for 10 hours. Breakfast may be served to the examinees after blood sampling if fasting was required.

Questionnaire to the parents

This record form is preferably filled in by the parents at home, in advance of the parents' examination (if any), and should be carefully checked for completeness and inconsistencies.

Identification data on the first page (including boxes 1–21) are completed in advance by the centre.

Centre code. A number assigned by WHO to each collaborating centre. This should be filled in by each centre and may be preprinted.

School or subgroup code. A two-digit number may be used by the centre for dividing the population into subgroups — according to schools or localities within the study area, for example. This code is allocated by the respective centre; its use is optional.

Name of child. Family name comes first, then other name(s), in the same way that the child figures at school.

Page 1 also contains instructions to the parents on how to fill in the questionnaire. The given text (see p. 129) is only an example. The centres are requested to review it carefully and to adapt it to the local conditions. Translation of the questionnaire into the national language requires great care.

When the parents appear for medical examination at the survey, it is recommended that the record be checked for completeness and possible inadequacies, in the presence of the parents.

Child's physical examination

Examination number. Enter (1) for first examination, (2) for first follow-up examination, etc.

Standing height. Measured using a scale fixed to the wall. Child standing without shoes, with feet at an angle of 45°, the back square against the wall and eyes looking straight ahead (top of the external auditory meatus is level with the external angle of the eye). Child asked to stand as upright as possible, with heels on the ground and the measuring square resting on the scalp and against the wall. Height measured once, to the nearest millimetre.

Weight. Measured once using a level balance, to the nearest 100 g, without shoes, in light undergarments. Child standing with both feet in the middle of the board and not allowed to stoop.

Skinfolds. Measured with a Harpenden caliper. The caliper should read 0 before measurement. A fold of skin is firmly picked up between the thumb and the forefinger, followed by tangential application of the Harpenden caliper on the skinfold. Reading is taken as soon as the pointer becomes stationary.

Left triceps skinfold is measured to the nearest millimetre, at the midpoint of the back of the upper arm, with the child standing, arm hanging relaxed.

Left subscapular skinfold is measured similarly to the triceps measurement, just below the angle of scapula.

Blood pressure. The random zero sphygmomanometer is recommended. Blood pressure is measured on the right arm, with the subject comfortably seated in a warm room. The arm has to rest on a soft support, with muscles relaxed. The individual to be examined should be seated for about 5 minutes prior to the examination; no vigorous exercise should have been carried out in the preceding 15 minutes.

Attention must be paid to the cuff used. A set of six cuffs of various sizes has to be available (see p. 126). The cuff is selected according to the child's arm: it should be the largest cuff whose bladder completely encircles the arm. Narrow and short cuffs give higher readings. The number of the cuff used should be noted on the record form (cuff code).

The pressure is measured twice, at an interval of 1–2 minutes. With both measurements, systolic and diastolic fourth and fifth phase (disappearance of Korotkoff sounds) are recorded. On both occasions, immediately following the blood pressure measurement, the pulse is counted for at least 30 seconds and heart rate per minute is recorded.

When reporting on results, details of the measurement situation should be described, such as zone temperature, number of people in the room, whether the measurement is done before or after venipuncture, etc.

Blood sampling. A blood sample is taken at the end of the examination. The operation depends on whether serum or plasma cholesterol only is determined, or whether glucose tolerance and triglyceride determinations are included as well; the latter are optional.

(a) Only serum and plasma cholesterol is determined. At the end of the examination a blood sample is drawn in the following way. The examinee is laid on a couch. A nurse or technician is seated on a stool. If the vein is not visible spontaneously, a soft elastic rubber band is applied for a short time. No attempt is made to perform venipuncture if the child is unwilling, or dizzy. Blood is drawn into a vacutainer, labelled, kept at room temperature, and sent to the laboratory on the same day. Not more than two venipunctures should be attempted in a child.

(b) Cholesterol, triglycerides, lipoproteins and glucose tolerance (optional). The examinees are told not to have anything to eat or drink except water during the preceding 10 hours. A 1 g/kg glucose solution is given in 200 ml of lemonade. The time of ingestion is noted on the record. Fifty-five minutes after the glucose load the examinee is laid on the couch, and preparations are

122

made for drawing the blood sample. In the sixtieth minute blood is drawn for serum cholesterol and triglyceride analysis; the tube is then removed and, via the same needle, blood is led to drip into a glass tube containing about 50 mg of sodium fluoride. The second tube is stoppered and gently rotated 10 times to mix the blood with the anticoagulant. Both tubes are labelled and then kept at 0°C until despatch to the laboratory, which should take place within 3 hours.

Assessment of sexual maturity. Sexual maturity in girls and boys is assessed according to the method described on pp. 127–128.

Smoking questionnaire. Children aged nine and older, and all adolescents, are asked questions about smoking. Each principal investigator will work out rules on how to ask the questions most appropriate to the local environment in order to obtain reliable answers. These questions may best be asked by a nurse, privately, encouraging the child to give a confidential answer without making the child feel guilty.

Physical activity. The assessment of physical activity is fraught with many methodological difficulties. A possible simple way of obtaining some information about schoolchildren's and adolescents' physical activity is based on the assumption that they have better school marks in physical education if they are physically more active, especially if engaged in sports and competitions. However, marks cannot be compared easily from school to school and investigators may have to work out their own criteria for rating of high, medium and poor activity.

Missing data. If a child has not been examined, or if any item is missing, the reason should be stated. A missing item may be coded later.

Pathological findings. If any finding is judged by the investigator to be pathological, requiring treatment (such as high blood pressure or hyperlipidaemia), the parents should be notified and the child referred to the family physician or a paediatrician.

Parents' physical examination

The same methods are applied as to their children.

Only adult-size blood pressure cuffs are used (cuff number 5 or 6).

A 12-lead resting ECG is taken. The machine should be checked for appropriate time constant. Each tracing must have a standardization mark. It is recommended that the tracings be mounted. Each tracing should be identified by full name and identity code, and date of examination. The tracings are coded according to the Minnesota Code.[a] Coding may be done by specially trained technicians.

---

[a] **Rose, G.A. & Blackburn, H.** *Cardiovascular survey methods.* Geneva, World Health Organization, 1968 (Monograph Series, No. 56).

Longitudinal study

As pointed out earlier, longitudinal study of the children and their parents is highly recommended.

It is recommended that, if possible, the children or a sample of them be re-examined each year, while the parents should be re-examined only three years later, i.e. in the fourth year of the study.

There are several questions to be answered by semi-longitudinal or longitudinal studies. These include the collection of data on tracking of serum cholesterol, blood pressure and other risk factors, changes in risk factors with age, changes in the population and within the group being studied, and information on the acceptability of intervention measures, and their effectiveness in reducing risk factors. There will need to be flexibility of study design as no single study can answer all those points. However, methods should conform to the WHO protocol to enable comparability of results from different studies. The same methods should be used throughout the study.

Dropouts — or a random sample of them — should be followed up. The reasons for dropping out should be ascertained and it should be made clear whether the results are likely to be influenced by possible selection due to dropout.

Training and standardization

Training and testing of observers for anthropometry

Training and testing of observers for anthropometry is carried out, prior to the onset of the survey, under the guidance of an experienced observer. The following steps are taken.

1.   Introductory lecture on examination techniques.

2.   Practical demonstration by a trained observer on the use of apparatus and procedural steps involved in anthropometry. Attention is paid to precise location of arm and scapula.

3.   Training of future observers, in turn, on 10 subjects, under the supervision of an experienced observer. Duplicate readings are taken and the means of trainees compared.

4.   Testing of observers, by comparing their results with those of the supervisor.

5.   Completion of training. Training is continued until the inter-observer differences cannot be further diminished.

After completion of training, observers with the best performance are assigned to anthropometry. It is felt that, while training for height and weight measurements is fairly easy, skinfold measurements present problems, particularly location of precise position and the manner of picking up the fold.

124

Training and testing of observers for blood pressure measurements

Training of observers for measuring blood pressure should preferably be organized by the principal investigator himself, or by his first assistant, in order to stress the importance of correct measurements. In a first series of measurements the future observers should take at least 20 measurements with an ordinary sphygmomanometer. They should record their own results and, in a second move, should be instructed to make an analysis of digit preference of their own readings.

Next, pairs of observers should listen to the same Korotkoff sounds through stethoscopes connected by a Y-tube. The findings should be recorded and compared.

Finally, the random zero sphygmomanometer (if used in the study) should be demonstrated and its use practised before starting the survey.

ECG coding standardization

Previous experience has shown that considerable effort needs to be invested in the standardization of ECG coding.

In the present study relatively few and mostly minor pathological ECG findings should be expected.

Standardization of laboratory methods

The choice of methods for cholesterol and triglyceride analysis is at the discretion of each investigator. If plasma cholesterorol is being measured, the type and concentration of anticoagulant being used may influence results, and these should, therefore, always be specified in a description of methodology. It is pointed out, however, that modifications of the Liebermann-Burchart method have been shown to give the most reliable results for serum cholesterol, and modifications of Zilversmit's method for serum triglycerides.

Choice of methods for lipoprotein analysis is at the discretion of each investigator. Where possible, methods should be standardized against an analytical ultracentrifuge method.

The standardization programme consists of four phases: familiarization and self-evaluation, short-term blind evaluation, standardization, and surveillance. Samples are shipped from the reference laboratory to the individual laboratories and their results are confidentially evaluated; reports are sent to each laboratory at defined intervals. However, the standardization programme does not replace normal internal quality control, to be carried out in every biochemical laboratory; on the contrary, interval quality control has to be reinforced.

Glucose standardization should be achieved by an adjacent university biochemical laboratory.

Appendix 1. Instruments for measuring blood pressure

The random zero sphygmomanometer is used, as described by B.M. Wright &
C.F. Dore: *Lancet*, **1**: 337–338 (1975).

Standard cuffs for measurements on children are described by M. Long
et al.: *Archives of disease in childhood*, **46**: 636–670 (1971). The dimensions
are as follows.

Cuff no.	Width (cm)	Length (cm)
1	2.5	10.0
2	5.0	10.0
3	7.5	15.0
4	10.0	19.0
5	12.5	23.0

The sixth cuff (14 × 28 cm) should be available.

<h1 style="text-align:center">Appendix 2. Assessment of sexual maturity[a]</h1>

Breast development in girls

The development of the mammae can be divided into five stages:

Stage 1: Pre-adolescent: elevation of papilla only.

Stage 2: Breast bud stage: elevation of breast and papilla as small mound. Enlargement of areolar diameter.

Stage 3: Further enlargement and elevation of breast and areola, with no separation of their contours.

Stage 4: Projection of areola and papilla to form a secondary mount above the level of the breast.

Stage 5: Mature stage: projection of papilla only, due to recession of the areola to the general contour of the breast.

Genital development in boys

The development of the external genitalia can be differentiated in five stages:

Stage 1: Pre-adolescent: testes, scrotum and penis are of about the same size and proportion as in early childhood.

Stage 2: Enlargement of scrotum and of testes. The skin of the scrotum reddens and changes in texture. Little or no enlargement of penis at this stage.

Stage 3: Enlargement of penis, which occurs at first mainly in length. Further growth of testes and scrotum.

Stage 4: Increased size of penis with growth in breadth and development of glands. Further enlargement of testes and scrotum; increased darkening of scrotal skin.

Stage 5: Genitalia adult in size and shape. No further enlargement takes place after stage 5 is reached; it seems, on the contrary, that the penis size decreases slightly from the immediately post-adolescent peak.

---

[a] From **Tanner, J.M.** *Growth at adolescence*. Oxford, Blackwell, 1962.

Pubic hair stages for girls and boys

Stage 1:   Pre-adolescent: the vellus over the pubes is not further developed than that over the abdominal wall, i.e. no pubic hair.

Stage 2:   Sparse growth of long, slightly pigmented downy hair, straight or only slightly curled, appearing chiefly at the base of the penis or along the labia.

Stage 3:   Considerably darker, coarser and more curled. The hair spreads sparsely over the junction of the pubes.

Stage 4:   Hair now resembles adult in type, but the area covered by it is still considerably smaller than in the adult. No spread to the medial surface of the thighs.

Stage 5:   Adult in quantity and type with distribution of the horizontal (or classically "feminine") pattern. Spread to medial surface of thighs but not up *linea alba* or elsewhere above the base of the inverse triangle.

Good lighting is essential for arriving at a correct appraisal of initial pubic hair.

Menarche

The inquiry into menarche takes place according to the so-called *status quo* method, by means of the question "Have you started your periods yet?" or something to that effect. The answer is recorded as "yes" or "no". If the examiner sees fit not to put this question for any reason whatever, this is also placed on record.

Appendix 3. Protocol for study of atherosclerosis precursors in children

STUDY OF ATHEROSCLEROSIS PRECURSORS
IN CHILDREN   1-4 ☐☐☐☐

QUESTIONNAIRE TO THE PARENTS   5 ☐

6- 8   Centre: _______________________________   ☐☐☐

9-10   School or subgroup: _________________   ☐☐

11-13 Name of child: ___________________________   ☐☐☐
                  Family name   First name(s)   Child's no.

       Address: ___________________________________

14   Sex   Male ☐1   Female ☐2   15-16   Age at last birthday ☐☐

17-22 Date of birth   ☐☐   ☐☐   19 ☐☐
                        day   month   year

INSTRUCTIONS TO THE PARENTS ON HOW
TO FILL IN THE ATTACHED QUESTIONNAIRE

Please read this questionnaire first, then start answering the questions. Kindly answer *all* questions by putting the mark X with a black pencil into the appropriate box. For instance:

Do you smoke cigarettes?   Yes ☐1   Never ☐2   Yes, but stopped ☐3

To some questions, the answer should be a number. For instance:

                                    day   month   year
Date of completing the questionnaire ☐☐   ☐☐   19 ☐☐

How many rooms are there in your house?
(If nine or more, enter 9) (including kitchen,
but excluding bathroom)   ☐

Boxes with broken lines will be filled in later, but please answer the questions verbally, according to your best knowledge. For instance:

Has your child ever had any serious disease?   Yes ☐1   No ☐2

If yes, please describe:

. . . .   ICD ☐☐☐

. . . .   ICD ☐☐☐

Thank you for your cooperation.

Date of completing the questionnaire ☐☐ ☐☐ 19☐☐   23-28

How many rooms are there in your household?
(If nine or more, enter 9) (including kitchen, but excluding bathroom)   ☐ 29

How many persons, including this child, usually live in your household?
(If nine or more, enter 9)   ☐ 30

Concerning the child

Has your child ever had any serious disease?   Yes ☐1   No ☐2   31

If yes, please describe:

. . . . ICD   ☐☐☐ 32-34

. . . . ICD   ☐☐☐ 35-37

Has your child ever been admitted to a hospital?   Yes ☐1   No ☐2   38

If yes, for what reasons?

. . . . ICD   ☐☐☐ 39-41

. . . . ICD   ☐☐☐ 42-44

Do you think that your child
smokes cigarettes?   Yes ☐1   No ☐2   Don't know ☐3   45

If yes, how many cigarettes per day?

1-4 ☐1   5-9 ☐2   10-14 ☐3   15-19 ☐4

20 or more ☐5   Don't know ☐9   46

Concerning the father of the child

Year of birth   19 ☐☐   If not alive, year of death   19 ☐☐   47-50

Cause of death . . . . ICD   ☐☐☐ 51-53

If alive, is the father living in the household?   Yes ☐1   No ☐2   54

The remainder of the questions relating to the father should only be answered if
the father is living in the household

Is this child yours by birth?   Yes ☐1   No ☐2   55

What is the level of your
school education?   Primary ☐1   Secondary ☐2   Higher ☐3   56

What is your primary occupation? . . . . Code   ☐☐ 57-58

Have you ever suffered from any of the following?

Heart attack	Yes ☐ 1	No ☐ 2	Don't know ☐ 3	59
Other heart disease	Yes ☐ 1	No ☐ 2	Don't know ☐ 3	60
High blood pressure	Yes ☐ 1	No ☐ 2	Don't know ☐ 3	61
Stroke	Yes ☐ 1	No ☐ 2	Don't know ☐ 3	62
Diabetes	Yes ☐ 1	No ☐ 2	Don't know ☐ 3	63
Any other serious illnesses?	Yes ☐ 1	No ☐ 2	Don't know ☐ 3	64

If yes, what illnesses?

. . . .   ICD   ☐☐☐ 65–67

. . . .   ICD   ☐☐☐ 68–70

. . . .   ICD   ☐☐☐ 71–73

Smoking habits:

	Yes	Never	Yes, but stopped		
Do you smoke cigarettes?	☐ 1	☐ 2	☐ 3	If yes, how many per day?	☐☐ 74–76
Do you smoke cigars?	☐ 1	☐ 2	☐ 3	If yes, how many per day?	☐☐ 77–79
Do you smoke pipes?	☐ 1	☐ 2	☐ 3	If yes, how many per day?	☐☐ 80–82

Concerning the father of the father

Is your father alive?   Yes ☐ 1   No ☐ 2   If no, at what age did he die? ☐☐ 83–85

Cause of death . . . .   ICD   ☐☐☐ 86–88

Has he, or had he, ever suffered from any of the following?

Heart attack	Yes ☐ 1	No ☐ 2	Don't know ☐ 3	89
Other heart disease	Yes ☐ 1	No ☐ 2	Don't know ☐ 3	90
High blood pressure	Yes ☐ 1	No ☐ 2	Don't know ☐ 3	91
Stroke	Yes ☐ 1	No ☐ 2	Don't know ☐ 3	92
Diabetes	Yes ☐ 1	No ☐ 2	Don't know ☐ 3	93
Any other serious illnesses?	Yes ☐ 1	No ☐ 2	Don't know ☐ 3	94

If yes, what illnesses?

. . . .   ICD |_|_|_| 95–97

. . . .   ICD |_|_|_| 98–100

Does he, or did he, smoke?   Heavily ☐ 1   Moderately ☐ 2   Never ☐ 3   101

Concerning the mother of the father

Is your mother alive?   Yes ☐ 1   No ☐ 2   If no, at what age did she die? ☐☐ 102–104

Cause of death . . . .   ICD |_|_|_| 105–107

Has she, or had she, ever suffered from any of the following?

Heart attack	Yes ☐ 1	No ☐ 2	Don't know ☐ 3	108
Other heart disease	Yes ☐ 1	No ☐ 2	Don't know ☐ 3	109
High blood pressure	Yes ☐ 1	No ☐ 2	Don't know ☐ 3	110
Stroke	Yes ☐ 1	No ☐ 2	Don't know ☐ 3	111
Diabetes	Yes ☐ 1	No ☐ 2	Don't know ☐ 3	112
Any other serious illnesses	Yes ☐ 1	No ☐ 2	Don't know ☐ 3	113

If yes, what illnesses?

. . . .   ICD |_|_|_| 114–116

. . . .   ICD |_|_|_| 117–119

Does she, or did she, smoke?   Heavily ☐ 1   Moderately ☐ 2   Never ☐ 3   120

132

Year of birth   19 ☐☐   If not alive, year of death   19 ☐☐   121–124

Cause of death . . . .   ICD   ⌐ I I ⌐   125–127

If alive, is the mother living in the household?   Yes ☐ 1   No ☐ 2   128

The remainder of the questions relating to the mother should only be answered if
the mother is living in the household

Is this child yours by birth?   Yes ☐ 1   No ☐ 2   129

What is the level of your
school education?   Primary ☐ 1   Secondary ☐ 2   Higher ☐ 3   130

What is your primary occupation?   . . . .   Code   ⌐ I ⌐ 131–132

Do you take
contraceptive pills?   Regularly ☐ 1   Irregularly ☐ 2   No ☐ 3   133

Have you ever suffered from any of the following?

Heart attack   Yes ☐ 1   No ☐ 2   Don't know ☐ 3   134

Other heart
disease   Yes ☐ 1   No ☐ 2   Don't know ☐ 3   135

High blood
pressure   Yes ☐ 1   No ☐ 2   Don't know ☐ 3   136

Stroke   Yes ☐ 1   No ☐ 2   Don't know ☐ 3   137

Diabetes   Yes ☐ 1   No ☐ 2   Don't know ☐ 3   138

Any other serious
illnesses?   Yes ☐ 1   No ☐ 2   Don't know ☐ 3   139

If yes, what illnesses?

. . . .   ICD   ⌐ I I ⌐ 140–142

. . . .   ICD   ⌐ I I ⌐ 143–145

. . . .   ICD   ⌐ I I ⌐ 146–148

Smoking habits:

	Yes	Never	Yes, but stopped		

Do you smoke cigarettes? ☐ 1 ☐ 2 ☐ 3   If yes, how many per day? ☐☐ 149–151

Do you smoke cigars? ☐ 1 ☐ 2 ☐ 3   If yes, how many per day? ☐☐ 152–154

Do you smoke pipes? ☐ 1 ☐ 2 ☐ 3   If yes, how many per day? ☐☐ 155–157

Concerning the father of the mother

Is your father alive?   Yes ☐ 1   No ☐ 2   If no, at what age did he die? ☐☐ 158–160

Cause of death . . . . ICD ☐☐☐ 161–163

Has he, or had he, ever suffered from any of the following?

Heart attack   Yes ☐ 1   No ☐ 2   Don't know ☐ 3   164

Other heart disease   Yes ☐ 1   No ☐ 2   Don't know ☐ 3   165

High blood pressure   Yes ☐ 1   No ☐ 2   Don't know ☐ 3   166

Stroke   Yes ☐ 1   No ☐ 2   Don't know ☐ 3   167

Diabetes   Yes ☐ 1   No ☐ 2   Don't know ☐ 3   168

Any other serious illnesses?   Yes ☐ 1   No ☐ 2   Don't know ☐ 3   169

If yes, what illnesses?

. . . . ICD ☐☐☐ 170–172

. . . . ICD ☐☐☐ 173–175

Does he, or did he, smoke?   Heavily ☐ 1   Moderately ☐ 2   Never ☐ 3   176

Concerning the mother of the mother

Is your mother alive?   Yes ☐ 1   No ☐ 2   If no, at what age did she die? ☐☐ 177–179

Cause of death . . . .   ICD |_ _|_ _|_ _| 180–182

Has she, or had she, ever suffered from any of the following?

Heart attack   Yes ☐ 1   No ☐ 2   Don't know ☐ 3   183

Other heart disease   Yes ☐ 1   No ☐ 2   Don't know ☐ 3   184

High blood pressure   Yes ☐ 1   No ☐ 2   Don't know ☐ 3   185

Stroke   Yes ☐ 1   No ☐ 2   Don't know ☐ 3   186

Diabetes   Yes ☐ 1   No ☐ 2   Don't know ☐ 3   187

Any other serious illnesses?   Yes ☐ 1   No ☐ 2   Don't know ☐ 3   188

If yes, what illnesses?

. . . .   ICD |_ _|_ _|_ _| 189–191

. . . .   ICD |_ _|_ _|_ _| 192–194

Does she, or did she, smoke?   Heavily ☐ 1   Moderately ☐ 2   Never ☐ 3   195

WHO STUDY OF ATHEROSCLEROSIS PRECURSORS IN CHILDREN

1–4 ☐☐☐☐

PARENT'S PHYSICAL EXAMINATION

5 ☐

6–8 Centre: ☐☐☐   9–10 School or subgroup: ☐☐   11–13 Child's number: ☐☐☐

Name of parent:

Family name   First name(s)

14 Sex: Male ☐ 1   Female ☐ 2   15–16 Age at last birthday ☐☐

135

If parent has already been examined, because there is another child in this study, please *fill in only* the next two items

17–18 School or subgroup: ☐

19–21 Child's number: ☐

---

22 Examination number:

23–28 Date of examination: ☐☐ ☐☐ 19 ☐☐
day · month · year

29–32 Standing height: ☐☐☐ ☐ cm

33–36 Body weight: ☐☐☐ ☐ kg

Skinfold:

	1st reading	2nd reading
37–40 Triceps	☐☐☐ mm	☐☐☐ mm
41–44 Subscapular	☐☐☐ mm	☐☐☐ mm

Blood pressure:

45 Cuff code ☐

Systolic

	1st reading	2nd reading
Random-zero	☐☐☐	☐☐☐
Zero-correction	☐☐☐	☐☐☐
46–51 Corrected value	☐☐☐ mmHg	☐☐☐ mmHg

Diastolic

	1st reading	2nd reading
Random-zero	☐☐☐	☐☐☐
Zero-correction	☐☐☐	☐☐☐
52–57 Corrected value	☐☐☐ mmHg	☐☐☐ mmHg
58–63 Heart-rate/minute	☐☐☐	☐☐☐

64–76 ECG:	1.1	1.2	1.3	2	3	4	5	6	7	8	9	9.4	9.8

Minnesota Code

Blood sampling:

77   Has the parent eaten in the last 10 hours?   Yes ☐ 1   No ☐ 2

78–80 Serum cholesterol   ☐☐☐ mg/dl

81–83 Serum triglyceride (fasting)   ☐☐☐.☐ g/l

84–86 Glucose tolerance (fasting)   ☐☐☐ mg/dl

87   Blood group (optional)   ☐ 1   ☐ 2   ☐ 3   ☐ 4   ☐ 5   ☐ 6

         O   A₁   A₂   B   A₁B   A₂B

---

88   If parent has not been examined, state reasons:

. . . . ☐

WHO STUDY OF ATHEROSCLEROSIS PRECURSORS IN CHILDREN

1–4 ☐☐☐☐

CHILD'S PHYSICAL EXAMINATION

5 ☐

6– 8 Centre: _______________________________ ☐☐☐

9–10 School or subgroup: _______________________ ☐☐

11–13 Name of child: ___________________________ ☐☐☐

         Family name   First name(s)

Address: ___________________________________

14 Sex: Male ☐ 1   Female ☐ 2   15–16 Age at last birthday ☐☐

17–22 Date of birth: ☐☐ ☐☐   19 ☐☐

         day   month   year

---

23 Examination number: ☐

24–29 Date of examination: ☐☐ ☐☐   19 ☐☐

         day   month   year

30–33 Standing height: ☐☐☐ ☐ cm

34–36 Body weight: ☐☐☐ ☐ kg

Skinfold: 1st reading   2nd reading

37–40 Triceps   ☐☐☐ mm   ☐☐☐ mm

41–44 Subscapular   ☐☐☐ mm   ☐☐☐ mm

Blood pressure:

45 Cuff code ☐

Systolic	1st reading	2nd reading
Random-zero	☐☐☐	☐☐☐
Zero-correction	☐☐☐	☐☐☐
46–51 Corrected value	☐☐☐ mmHg	☐☐☐ mmHg

Diastolic		
Random-zero	☐☐☐	☐☐☐
Zero-correction	☐☐☐	☐☐☐
52–57 Corrected value	☐☐☐ mmHg	☐☐☐ mmHg
58–63 Heart-rate/minute	☐☐☐	☐☐☐

64–76 ECG: (at age 15 and over)	1.1	1.2	1.3	2	3	4	5	6	7	8	9	9.4	9.8

Minnesota Code

Blood sampling:

77 Has the child eaten in the last 10 hours?   Yes ☐ 1   No ☐ 2

78–80 Serum cholesterol   ☐☐☐ mg/dl

81–83 Serum triglyceride (fasting)   ☐☐☐ ☐ g/l

84–86 Glucose tolerance (fasting)   ☐☐☐ mg/dl

87 Blood group (optional)

☐ 1   ☐ 2   ☐ 3   ☐ 4   ☐ 5   ☐ 6
O A_1 A_2 B A_1 B A_2 B

Sexual maturity:

88 Genital development in boys or breast development in girls   ☐

89 Development of pubic hairs in both sexes   ☐

90 Menarche in girls   Yes ☐ 1   No ☐ 2   Question not asked   ☐

Smoking habits:

91   Child is too young to be asked   ☐ 1

92   Do you smoke?   Yes ☐ 1   No ☐ 2

93-94   How old were you when you started smoking?   ☐ years

95-96   How many cigarettes do you smoke per day?

97   Do you smoke every day?   Yes ☐ 1   No ☐ 2

98   Although you do not smoke, have you ever smoked or lit a cigarette?   Yes ☐ 1   No ☐ 2

Physical activity:

99   How active are you physically?   Very active ☐ 1   Fairly active ☐ 2   Rather inactive ☐ 3   Not applicable ☐ 4

---

100   If child has not been examined, state reason:

. . . . ☐
